CHILDBEARING AFTER 35

The Risks and The Rewards

by Dr. Francesca C. Fay and Kathy S. Smith

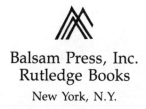

Balsam Press, Inc.
Rutledge Books
New York, N.Y.

AUTHORS' NOTE

While both of us have given birth twice, only Francesca has done so over 35, so it is her experience of childbearing at 36 and 40 that are referred to in the first person singular—"I," "my," and so on—in the text.

Copyright © 1985 by Balsam Press, Inc.
All rights reserved. No part of this work may be
reproduced or transmitted in any form or by any means
without written permission.

Distributed by Kampmann & Company
9 East 40th Street
New York, New York 10016

Jacket photograph by Dennis Hallinan/FPG International

Library of Congress Cataloging in Publication Data
Fay, Francesca C.
   Childbearing after 35.

   1. Pregnancy in middle age. 2. Childbirth. I. Smith,
Kathy S. (Kathy Sammis) II. Title. III. Title:
Childbearing after thirty-five
RG556.6.F39   1985   618.2   85-3906
ISBN 0-917439-05-8

Editor: Jennifer Weis
Art Director: Allan Mogel
Executive Editor: Barbara Krohn

Manufactured in the United States of America

DEDICATION

To my husband, Leon, and my children, Ashley and Jamie.—F.F.

To my mother, an over-30 childbearer herself.—K.S.

ACKNOWLEDGEMENTS

We are grateful for the time and knowledge shared with us by the following people: Jefrey Arlen, M.D., Associate Director, Family Practice Residency Program, St. Mary's Medical Center, Evansville, Indiana; Dwight Cruikshank, M.D., Director, Maternal-Fetal Medicine, Medical College of Virginia Hospital, Richmond, Virginia; Edward M. Kloza, M.S., Administrative Director, Clinical Genetics Division, Foundation for Blood Research, Scarborough, Maine; Jeffrey M. Saffer, M.D., Family Practitioner, Cape Elizabeth, Maine; Joan Tremblay, R.N., Ob-Gyn Nurse Practitioner, Dartmouth-Mary Hitchcock Medical Center, Hanover, New Hampshire; our enthusiastic editor, Jennifer Weis; and the many women we interviewed who gladly shared their experiences of over-35 childbearing with us.

Table of Contents

CHAPTER 1

OVER 35 AND WANTING A BABY— YOU'RE NOT ALONE

A significant change is occurring in childbearing in the United States. It began in the 1970's and continues into the 1980's. Pregnant women are becoming older. Only 10 to 15 years ago, obstetricians viewed first-time mothers over 30 with jaundiced eyes, expecting them to have serious obstetrical problems and, often, babies with birth defects. The medical term for such a woman was (and is) "elderly primigravida." Yet today, it is a rare obstetrician who does not have a number of patients over 30, over 35, even over 40, who are preparing for their first child. In fact, pregnancy for women in their early 30's has become commonplace and medically unexceptional, and has brought with it acceptance of pregnancy for women over 35.

The good news is that everything is coming together to make having a baby after 35 safer, and therefore, more often done. If you've waited until now and worried whether it isn't too late, read on and learn what you can do to maximize your chances of getting pregnant in the first place—for the decreased fertility of older women is one of the biggest problems would-be parents encounter—and learn what you can do to make yourself optimally fit and ready to conceive, carry and deliver a healthy baby despite being over 35.

There are some definite risks involved, such as bearing a child with Down's syndrome, but medical tests have become safer and more sophisticated so that you can find out before you have your baby whether she or he will be normal and healthy, and if not, the choice will be yours whether to continue the pregnancy or not. The advances of medical technology that make all this possible, coupled with some changes in the role of women and men today, make a new book summarizing these developments important.

Birth Postponement: Who Chooses It

There really are more older mothers today, and they have become highly visible. The *Time* magazine cover story of February 22, 1982, was "The New Baby Bloom" and featured a cover photo of actress Jaclyn Smith, seven months pregnant at the age of 35. Other actresses who are also recent "elderly primigravidas" include Jill Clayburgh (38 when she gave birth), Faye Dunaway (41), Ursula Andress (45), Paula Prentiss (36—and then she had a second), and Farrah Fawcett (37). Writers Erica Jong and Nora Ephron waited until after 35 to become mothers. So did journalist Sally Quinn, whose first child was born when she was 40.

It's not just celebrities who are having babies later in life. I've spoken with a number of women in everyday life who became mothers after 35, and who typify the new older mothers. A woman who has her first child in her mid 30's is likely to have a college education and live in an urban area. She did not marry young. She has a well-paying job and, since her salary is comparable to her husband's, the family income is well above average. She and her spouse prepare thoroughly for the pregnancy and delivery. She is physically fit, weight conscious, and exercises regularly.

Census Bureau figures reflect the trend. While the first-birth rate for women under 25 has fallen, that rate has risen steadily for women between 30 and 39. (The first-birth rate for women 40 to 44 has stayed the same.) The largest increase in rate has been for women 35 to 39; they registered an astonishing 300% gain from 1973 to 1983 in first births, even though, at this age, their fertility was declining. During the same period, women from 30 to 34 also experienced a dramatic first-birth rate increase of 97%. Even women 25 to 29 upped their first-birth rate by 33%, although that rate then fell by 1% between 1981 and 1982.

While most of the births in the seventies and early eighties were to mothers under 30, the figures for women over 30 do show a dramatic rise, especially when expressed in numbers of babies born. Women aged 35 to 39 had 115,409 live births in 1975; by 1980 they gave birth to 140,793 babies, with the 1983 figure up to 225,000. Comparable numbers for women 30 to 34 are 370,000 in 1973 and 658,000 for 1983. First-time mothers aged 35 to 39 totalled 9,639 in 1973. In the year from June 1982 to June 1983 women in this age group registered more than 42,500 first births.

This increase in total births for women in their 30's has been accompanied by a steady rise in the percentage of those births that produce a first child. In 1970, only 6½% of births to women 35 to 39 years old produced a first child, while nearly half of those births represented a fifth child or more. By 1983, the percentage of first births to women in this age group was close to 20%, while the proportion of fifth or higher births has plummeted.

Birth Postponement Patterns

Why is this happening? The reasons for the older-parenthood phenomenon are intertwined. Socioeconomic factors have joined medical/technological ones; as it has become safer and surer to give birth at an older age, social and economic factors have made it advantageous to wait till later to have a baby.

First, of course, women can now choose when—and if—to have babies. It's easy for those of us born after 1940 to forget that there was no safe, simple, and really effective method of contraception until 1960, the year the Pill became commonly available. With the advent of the birth-control pill, followed by the IUD, women for the first time in history could control their childbearing to suit their own priorities. And they did. The U.S. birth rate dropped steadily throughout the sixties, hitting a low in 1976. Legalized abortion made it even more possible to make childbearing a choice.

The activism of the sixties also encouraged young women not to have children. Zero population growth was urged as a social obligation. Many young people felt it unfair to bring a child into a world whose survival was threatened by nuclear annihilation, environmental poisoning, and resource shortage. These young people are now reaching their mid 30's and re-thinking their choices on childbearing.

The strong women's movement of the 1970's encouraged each woman to shape her own identity, to think of herself in terms of her own unique individuality rather than to define herself as a wife, as a mother. Once pregnancy was no longer accepted as the near-inevitable result of marriage and/or sexual activity, women postponed pregnancy to develop other aspects of their lives: education, career, marriage without motherhood. Young women completing high school and college began to view their 20's as a time to enrich themselves, to grow and mature and achieve.

Contraception, sixties activism, and feminism, then, changed the way women lived and thought about themselves. Like young men, young women now aspire to well-paying, interesting, and challenging jobs, many of which require advanced education and/or training followed by a period of career-ladder climbing. Marriage and parenthood don't necessarily fit easily into this self-absorbing time.

Population surveys confirm that many better educated women in their 20's now delay parenthood and that older first-time mothers are much better educated today than they were 10 or 15 years ago. The vast majority have at least one year of college behind them, and many are college graduates. Furthermore, compared with their nonemployed sisters, women who work or worked marry later (which means later childbearing), expect and have fewer children, and allow more time between pregnancies. Wives who work after marriage wait longer before having a first child. And, of course, there are ever-increasing numbers of women in the labor force, meaning an ever-increasing number of women who exhibit this altered pattern of childbearing.

Starting in 1970 there has been a steady and large growth in the number of women over 25 who have no children. In 1970, 14% of white women were childless under age 30; in 1980, the figure was 27%. By 1983, 58% of American women under the age of 30 were childless. At the same time, the number of women in their late 20's and 30's has mushroomed. The post-World War II baby boom children are maturing. In the 10-year span from 1970 to 1980, the proportion of women over 30 in the population increased by more than 43%. The Census Bureau expects the number of women 35 to 44 to increase by 42% between 1980 and 1990. The increased number of women in their early 30's has combined with the increased childlessness to produce an ever-growing population of women who are "at risk" of having a first child in their 30's.

My life certainly followed this new pattern. After I graduated from college, I continued my studies and at the same time began my career. By the time I had earned three advanced degrees, I had also amassed a solid practical background in nursing and nursing education. I didn't marry while I was doing all this—it's hard to imagine having had the time to work on establishing a marriage then! I was 34 when I finally did marry, and 36 by the time I had my first child—a statistically typical older, well-educated, career-oriented first-time mother.

Other realities affected my childbearing patterns, as they have hundreds of thousands of other women. As in my case, most U.S. households now include two wage earners, as a matter of necessity. Since a woman is probably going to have to work, it makes sense for her to get the background she needs to lift her out of the traditionally low-paying "women's" jobs. If she's going to work like a man, she wants to earn like a man— and men don't drop out to raise children just as they're beginning to scale the career ladder. Young couples are also conscious of the cost of a child today. Giving birth and raising a child are very expensive. Prudence suggests delaying childbirth until a measure of financial security is attained.

Also, women no longer expect marriage to equal support for life. Marriage does not endure as it once did, as a glance at the mushrooming divorce rate shows, and in the event of divorce, alimony and child support are no longer necessarily forthcoming. A woman knows that if she chooses childrearing over career building, she may one day be forced to support herself and those children, alone, with few marketable skills, and those leading only to low-paying jobs. Starting a career at 25 or older is likely to be a lot harder than starting a family at that age. So the very real possibility of divorce is a potent factor is delaying childbearing. Even women with well-established careers often will not rush into pregnancy right after marriage. They want time to test the stability of the marriage first.

There is another reason why the high rate of divorce creates older parents. People who divorce in their 20's may not have had any children. By the time they remarry (and most divorced people do), they may be in their early or mid 30's. Only now does the woman have her first child. Or, although she already has a child, she and her second husband decide to have a child together. In either case, the new mother is likely to be in her mid 30's.

Approaching or reaching the age of 35 brings new factors

into play for the woman who has delayed childbearing until now. The famous biological time clock is ticking very loudly at this point. The initial faint sounds are heard at 30, when many women first begin thinking about having a child, sometime in the coming 5 to 10 years. By 35, a woman is most aware that her reproductive years will not last indefinitely. After 35, the childbirth-risk quotient must also be considered seriously. The pressure is on to make a conscious decision, either to begin childbearing or to have that one last child.

This dilemma has become widespread enough to be depicted on network TV. In a 1984 episode of *Cagney and Lacey*, 38-year-old Chris Cagney, an unmarried police detective, thought she was pregnant. When she found out she was not, the impact hit her. She didn't want a baby just then, but how much longer did she have? Angry that she couldn't "do a damn thing about" the biological clock, she railed at men's ability to have babies at 60, 70, 80.

Age 35 tends to be a time of upheaval for all women, mothers and nonmothers alike. It is likely to be the midlife crisis period, more often experienced by men at 40, when a person reexamines and reassesses her life, her current situation. For the career person, it can be a time when personal needs and desires become more important than or as important as career goals, especially personal goals that were put aside until now. A woman who has postponed parenthood or delayed the birth of another child may well find herself drawn to the concept now.

While the mid-30's woman wrestles with her midlife crisis and copes with the approaching end of her childbearing years, another twist may confront her. Her doctor may recommend that she stop taking the Pill because of an increasing risk of vascular problems, especially if she smokes. The chart which follows graphically depicts the age-related hazards of Pill use. A woman who for years has relied on the Pill and now must choose an alternate form of contraception may well decide that this is the appropriate time to become pregnant, or at least the time to try for a while.

Postponed childbearing is helped along by the recent change in society's attitude toward the single-child family, which has become acceptable. While it is acknowledged that an

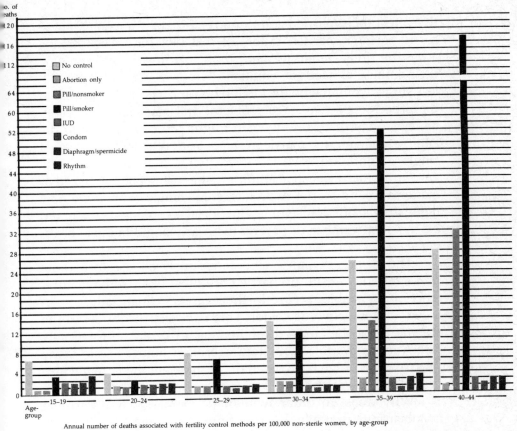

Annual number of deaths associated with fertility control methods per 100,000 non-sterile women, by age-group

[Source: Howard W. Ory, "Mortality Associated with Fertility and Fertility Control: 1983," Reprinted with permission from *Family Planning Perspectives*, 15:2 (March/April 1983), p. 58.]

only child can be spoiled and self-centered, it is also agreed that he or she is likely to be a high achiever, many of whom earn quite a bit more money than average later in life. Women who do not feel pressured to have more than one child can delay their sole pregnancy for a number of years; they don't need to get their first pregnancy underway in order to allow time for subsequent childbearing.

Single Parenthood

The late-pregnancy trend also involves single, unpartnered women, who are influenced by the same socioeconomic forces that affect their married counterparts. Single women are just as aware as their married sisters of that biological clock ticking away the time. Single women, too, turn inward and examine their emotional needs at "midlife." Ten or 15 years ago, a childless single woman who decided to become a parent approached the process as a two-stage problem: first marriage, then pregnancy. Today that same woman might proceed directly to the latter, eschewing the marriage stage. Society's strictures against single parenthood have loosened; while a single parent will encounter many negative attitudes, she will not be ostracized or made to wear a scarlet A. In fact, some single women are now requesting artificial insemination. Social acceptance is furthered by the vast number of parents who are single because of divorce.

Those single women who consciously choose to become pregnant and remain unmarried are most likely to be mature, emotionally stable, secure in their careers, financially advantaged—in other words, older. This is in sharp contrast to the stereotype of the "unwed mother" as an unstable, financially disadvantaged adolescent from a broken home. While many unpartnered pregnant women do fit the stereotype, many also fit the older woman's profile.

Why does an older woman deliberately choose single childbearing? Basically, because time is running out. She contemplates in great depth her desire to have a child, to commit herself fully to a relationship, and determines not to be denied this fulfillment by the fact that she has no long-term male partner. Deciding to continue the pregnancy, whether planned or unplanned, is very complex for a single woman, with resolution taking much longer than for partnered women. An over-35 prospective mother may well have had a prior abortion, and feel that if she has another she may be discarding her last chance at motherhood; she may feel ready and even eager, at last, to assume that role. Those women who do go ahead with the pregnancy generally do so on their own terms, regardless of the baby's father's reactions or future intentions.

Announcing the pregnancy, too, is more difficult for single than for partnered women. If the father is sure to urge abortion or the relatives sure to be horrified or dismayed, a woman will put off disclosing the happy news until it shows. Naturally, negative reactions produce stress and anxiety. However, single women interviewed by Virginia Peterson Tilden (*JOGN Nursing*, January/February 1983) reported that no stigma had been attached to their pregnancies by peers, health-care workers, or employers; only their parents had reacted negatively, and then only until the child was born, after which they became loving grandparents. Surprisingly, employers were concerned only about maternity-leave plans, just as they were with married workers.

The biggest drawback to single childbearing is the absence of an on-site, continuing support person. Expectant single mothers must consciously reach out to replace the support usually provided by a baby's father. In most cases they succeed, using friends, relatives, older children, health practitioners, and support groups. This was the conclusion of another study reported by Tilden (*Nursing Research*, March/April 1984), which found that single pregnant women do not have less emotional and informational support than partnered expectant mothers. However, they do have less tangible, or practical, support—a ride to the hospital at a moment's notice, for example. Women do feel stressed by single pregnancy, Tilden's study also found, but they do not suffer from more depression or lower self-esteem than partnered pregnant women.

Women choosing to become single mothers must consider legal aspects, a concern married women are free of. All of Tilden's interviewees, for example, had some concerns about relevant law. What last name is on the birth certificate? Is the father named on the certificate? Does the father have any rights to the child? Any obligations for support? Can a sister be named as legal guardian of the child rather than the father if the mother dies? Can the child inherit from the father's estate? What exactly are the legal consequences, immediate and future, of "illegitimacy"?

Single childbearing is a difficult but immensely rewarding experience. This is the conclusion of my close friend Nina, who at 40 has been a single mother for five years. Involved in a long-term relationship with a married man, Nina decided at 33 she wanted a child, someone who would "be there for her." Two years later she conceived and gave birth to a son, Justin. While Nina is psychologically very positive about single mothering, the lack of practical and financial support has, she admits, been difficult. When she experienced severe nausea and vomiting for the first five months of her pregnancy, she felt unable to use sick leave that would be needed after the baby's birth. When Justin was ill or up in the night, Nina was the sole caretaker and decision maker, and when babysitters or day-care providers became unreliable or used questionable judgment, Nina felt stressed in dealing with the situation alone. Nevertheless, the close and warm bond between her and her son makes Nina quite positive she has made the right choice. Single childbearing is not for everyone, but for those who do embrace it, the rewards more than outweigh the difficulties.

Advantages and Disadvantages of Older Parenthood

There are many reasons why women delay childbearing and don't complete their families before they're 35. But knowing why people choose to delay or extend parenthood is only part of the picture. What is the impact of that choice? What advantages and disadvantages do older parents experience?

Advantages

A woman having her first child at 35-plus is likely to be financially secure. The time an older expectant couple has had to accumulate savings to bridge any gaps in medical coverage and maternity benefits and to fund baby-equipment and baby-care purchases gives them a sizable advantage over young parents. An older mother's financial security is often matched by job security; her employer is likely to have a vested interest in her and therefore to accommodate her reasonable needs for maternity leave and time off.

That job security can also provide her with an emotional advantage. She may feel quite relaxed about pausing in her career for childraising and confident about her ability to return to the job market. A person who's worked for years knows that jobs can be boring, repetitive, and unfulfilling, and can weigh that in the balance when life at home with a small child begins to feel tedious.

Increased years bring increased maturity, along with realistic expectations, certainly advantages when dealing with the demands, quirks, stresses, and crises imposed by a child. An older person is more experienced and can be expected to have more knowledge of human nature and life's inconsistencies. Older parents have well-established adult identities, which won't be eroded by their baby. Very importantly, they've resolved their conflicts with their own parents, which frees them to accept the role of becoming a parent themselves. Over and over, the women I spoke with affirmed, "I know who I am now—it makes me a better parent."

Many older couples have had time to develop a close and comfortable understanding of the way they live and function together. This makes it easier to share the strains of childrearing. Older parents have also usually taken full advantage of their unencumbered state in their earlier years. They've traveled; vacationed; gone out to dinner, the theater, or the track whenever they wanted to and on the spur of the moment. They've socialized freely and frequently for years. By their mid 30's, they're not at all unwilling to slow down somewhat. Being realistic, they know that a baby is going to force a drastic slowdown in outside activities, but they also don't resent this as younger couples might. In all likelihood, they're ready for a new direction anyway. In the earliest, most time-consuming months of parenthood, they don't feel the anxiety so many young couples do that they're losing touch—permanently!— with the outside world; experience has shown them that people, places, and things will be pretty much the same out there from one month or season to the next.

An over-35 pregnancy is most often planned, or at least embraced gratefully after the fact. This produces a very positive attitude and a well-tended nine months. The older mother, especially the well-educated, financially secure one, usually initiates prenatal care early in pregnancy and consciously works at keeping herself and her developing baby in good health. This is obviously beneficial and gets parenthood off to an optimal start. Fitness, a good diet, and good prenatal care can also compensate for the physical and medical disadvantages an older woman theoretically has during pregnancy. The older father, too, usually follows the pregnancy closely, providing a high level of support for his partner.

When the baby arrives, the older parents continue to exhibit a very positive attitude. They often feel a great sense of accomplishment and fulfillment; they experience the baby as an enrichment of their lives. Many observers especially remark that older fathers involve themselves much more thoroughly in their children's care and development than do younger men, whether theirs are first children or not.

Older parents also report that being pregnant and having a young child makes them feel more youthful. Instead of being settled into mature, sedentary, adult pursuits, they're involved in Halloween costumes, nursery school outings, and Little League. They're kept up to date on Smurfs, Gremlins, and Cabbage Patch Kids. They experience holidays from a child's point of view and revive their own childhood feelings. They're involved in a younger world and so feel younger. Today's emphasis on fitness helps, too; people in their 40's, 50's, and 60's are more active and physically younger than in the past.

As older parenthood becomes more common, new parents over 35 are not necessarily going to feel like social oddballs. Most of the women I spoke with who had given birth in their late 30's and early 40's had worried about "being the oldest mother in the PTA or kindergarten." None had actually felt that way when the time came; each found a number of other mothers somewhere near her own age. Elaine, a 39-year-old resident of Manhattan, remarked that in her milieu, the 26-year-old with a toddler is the oddity; older mothers like herself are the norm. When 40-year-old Irene took her son to nursery school, she not only found many mothers in her age group but also found fathers who were much older, a result of second marriages that produced new children.

Few of these women had encountered adverse reactions from relatives, friends, co-workers, or society at large on account of their age. Anne, having her third child at 38, got some admonitions from her family about self-control and birth control, but the usual response was that of 35-year-old Laura's grandmother: "Finally, honey, finally." One woman and her husband, both 35, did overhear two teenage girls at a restaurant comment, "Gee, look at that cute baby with that old couple!" But the happy parents found the incident humorous rather than upsetting. Although there may be some concern about possible increased risk, the attitude today is overwhelmingly that becoming pregnant after 35 is simply normal.

Disadvantages

While becoming a parent over 35 has many pluses, there are minuses to consider as well. A woman who has worked hard to advance in her career may not be willing to disrupt that progress. Although millions of women have demonstrated that it is possible to pursue a career and also be a mother, it is unquestionably difficult and distracting to do so. A baby will interfere with total concentration on the job and with extended hours, travel, and work-related outside activities. There are also few role models for a career-woman mother to follow, other than her contemporaries. It's highly unlikely that her mother did what she's doing. A well-paid career woman also faces high "opportunity costs" of childbearing; staying home to care for a child means the loss of the opportunity to earn substantial sums. It's more expensive for her to take time off for childraising than for a lower-paid woman, so she may feel less justified in doing so.

Mid-30's couples are likely to have a stable, well-established lifestyle. Routines are comfortably set, and although they may be open to change, the introduction of a baby can be frighteningly disruptive. A childless couple over 35 has become accustomed to a one-on-one relationship. Socially and at work, they usually interact almost exclusively with adults. They're used to dealing with relatively mature, sensible, noninvasive individuals, not irrational, demanding, and dependent toddlers. The same can be true of an older couple whose other children are far from babyhood.

Over-35 parents may be the first of their friends to have a child. If so, the lost frequency and spontaneity of their social interactions can be difficult for those friends to understand and accept. The new parents' absorption with their child will likewise be baffling and boring to their childless peers. These over-35 parents will also be out of step with their friends whose children are finishing high school and going off to college. An older mother who's chosen to stay home with her baby, at least for a while, may feel socially isolated, cut off from her friends who aren't doing this or did it long ago.

Older parents, expectant or after the fact, also face questions not relevant to younger couples. Who asks a 25-year-old,

"Why did you decide to have a baby now?" Yet a 37-year-old may still expect to be quizzed, although this attitude is fading away with the increasing acceptance of older pregnancy. Avowed feminists may also encounter considerable self-doubt as well as challenges from others. If childbearing is a prime cause of female dependency and domination, aren't you contributing to the problem by becoming pregnant yourself? Aren't you falling into society's trap, selling out, becoming a Stepford Wife?

There are certain physical disadvantages to delaying pregnancy till 35 or later. Some risk factors do increase with age, although much can be done to minimize them—see Chapter 6. It will almost certainly be harder to get back into shape after delivery, just as it's harder to stay in shape, pregnant or not. Couples who don't start a family until after 35 may, because of fertility problems, pregnancy loss, or medical complications, be unable to have as many children as they would have wanted. They may even be unable to have any at all. Time does run out eventually for a woman, as discussed in Chapter 2.

Couples who have a child after 35 are tied down by child-rearing in their 40's and 50's, an age when other parents are often becoming liberated from that responsibility. (This can be offset by the freedom of unencumbered earlier years.) Parents who can pay during their 40's for their children's college education can then devote their 50's to preparing financially for retirement. Parents who are paying higher-education costs in their 50's have precious little left to put aside for retirement during those years. Their own parents may become a financial responsibility too at this time, creating a real economic nightmare. Sixty-year-old parents of college students may well ask themselves when they can ever retire!

Mixed Blessings

Couples contemplating delayed childbearing also wonder whether it will have a positive or negative impact on their children. They worry that, being older, they'll both look and seem different to their kids, whose friends will have noticeably younger parents. This is not likely to be a problem, however, since there are plenty of older parents around and since parents of any age are perceived as quite ancient by children. Kids notice the quality of their interaction with their parents, not their parents' ages. This can be less of a concern for prospective parents whose own parents were older when they were children, assuming a good parent–child relationship was established.

Nevertheless, a couple that is quite confident about caring for young children can find the concept of being over 50 and parenting teenagers positively daunting. Will they be flexible enough to tolerate the rebellion and irrationality of adolescence? Probably, if they've become typical older parents who are more patient and accepting of their children's behavior. Younger parents might be forced to deal with midlife crisis *and* teenagers simultaneously—truly daunting.

Over-35 parents may also worry about not being there for their children's major adult life events—college graduation, marriage, the birth of their children's children. Life expectancy, however, is constantly increasing. If a woman is 40 when her son is born, she can confidently expect to be healthy and not even retired when he finishes law school at 25 and marries at 30. She may, of course, have to wait till she's 75 before her son's first child is born.

Grandparent availability is a genuine concern for those who delay having children. If the present trend continues and their children also delay, they may be fairly old before they can enjoy becoming grandparents. Also, their own parents may be so old when the children are born that they lack the stamina or good health to interact as fully with the grandchildren as they would have done when they were younger. This would be a real deprivation for all three generations.

On the whole, couples who decide to have a child after 35 consider their choice very carefully. They weigh all these factors, the pluses and minuses, do what they can to overcome any disadvantages, and happily enjoy the advantages.

CHAPTER 2

GETTING PREGNANT

You're 36. You've put off pregnancy for years while you finished your graduate studies, advanced to a satisfying level in your career, traveled, enjoyed your evolving relationship with your mate. Now you've both decided it's time to have a baby. Cheerfully you discard all forms of contraception, apply yourself with relish to the task, and—nothing happens.

What's wrong? Your friend Emily seems to get pregnant every time she *looks* at her husband. Your sister-in-law postponed her first pregnancy till she was 39 and then conceived her child two months after she started trying. You've been at it for close to a year now with no results. What's wrong with you?

Recognizing Fertility Problems

Unfortunately, you've stumbled into what is probably the biggest hurdle you'll face in over-35 pregnancy: getting pregnant in the first place. A woman in her 30's is simply less fertile than a woman in her 20's. Female fertility peaks around age 24, followed by a gradual decline through the 30's and a rapid drop in the 40's. Male fertility also peaks in the 20's, but the subsequent decline is very gradual. A classic study by Alan F. Guttmacher did find that it took men over 35 three times as long as men under 25 to impregnate their wives in a six-month period. Still, even men in their 80's may be able to father children.

Both male and female factors contribute to infertility, which, incidentally, isn't the same as sterility; sterility is the absolute inability to reproduce, whereas infertility is a failure to conceive after a period of regular noncontraceptive intercourse.

Several age-related factors combine to affect female fertility. The older you are, the more time you have had to develop gynecological problems—fibroid tumors, endometriosis, scarring of the often very delicate reproductive organs. This can easily occur with no outward symptoms, so there is no indication that a fertility problem is developing. Also, ovulation patterns change with age. Long before menopause occurs, you usually begin to ovulate less frequently—you still bleed, but no egg has been released. This is called an "anovulatory" menstrual cycle. By the time you turn 40, 3 out of 12 cycles may be infertile; this increases to 7 out of 12 by the time you're 46. And when you do ovulate, the eggs may be released late; these eggs are often defective or can't be fertilized properly or, if fertilized, can't implant properly in the uterus—which results, sooner or later, in a spontaneous abortion. Age itself may affect the ability of the uterus to maintain a pregnancy, which aggravates the problem.

Added to all this is the fact that the older you are, the older your eggs are. Whereas a man produces fresh supplies of sperm continually throughout his reproductive life, a woman is born with all the eggs she will ever produce—about 400,000. Only about 400 of these will ever mature and be released for fertilization, and those with the greatest potential for fertilization are released earliest. The rest degenerate and die, or simply age. As they age, they're exposed to all the hazards of life— infections, drugs, radiation, pollutants. An older egg is more likely to be defective and not amenable to fertilization. Since sperm do not age in the same way, the effect of a man's age on sperm quality is much less direct and still a matter of speculation. Studies in this area are in their infancy.

These factors can affect a couple's ability to conceive a second child as well as a first. Pregnancy can be easily achieved on the first try but seem impossible on the next attempt. Why? The couple's fertility may be borderline, but they were lucky the first time. Their fertility may have changed—time has passed, and all the factors that affect fertility have had more time to come into play. Or they are perfectly fertile, but just on the wrong end of the pregnancy odds for now.

None of this is to say that you're sure to have trouble conceiving if you're over 35. You're not even *likely* to have trouble. You are, however, "at risk" for difficulty. And 15% of all U.S. couples—one out of seven—experience fertility disorders.

The problem is, if you wait until you're 35-plus to discontinue contraception, it may be a year before you decide you need help in conceiving. Now time is running short. Fertility treatments can take years, depending on the nature of the problem and, simply, on the odds. Many women neglect to allow for the possibility of delay in conception. One gynecologist linked this to today's demand for instant gratification, citing the number of women who consult him if they don't become pregnant within one month.

Failure to conceive, then, can come as quite a shock. *The New England Journal of Medicine* published a French fertility study on February 18, 1982, that showed a sharp decline in female fertility after age 30. The results were immediately challenged, especially since the women in the study were participating in artificial insemination and therefore presumably more likely to have had fertility problems to begin with. Most interesting, though, were the reactions in this country after the report was publicized in popular magazines and newspapers. *McCall's* (September 1982) wrote that women were very upset and very angry. *The New York Times* (February 25, 1982) uncovered feelings of panic and a sense of betrayal. Society has said it's okay to postpone pregnancy; society hasn't passed the word that there may be an infertility tradeoff involved.

Just what are your chances of achieving pregnancy? Clearly, they vary with age. The table below shows the odds a sexually active woman using no contraception has of becoming pregnant within one year at differing ages.

Age of Woman	% Conceiving after One Year
20–24	93
25–29	89
30–34	84
35–39	77

[Source: John Bongaarts, "Infertility after Age 30: A False Alarm," adapted with permission from the author and *Family Planning Perspectives*, 14:2 (March/April 1982).]

Many women who remain nonpregnant after 12 months may expect to conceive in the succeeding years. For example, among women of all ages, 80% can achieve pregnancy within one year; by the end of two years, the figure rises to 90%. Somewhat different age-related conception rates in artificial insemination are charted later in this chapter.

Another way of expressing this is to figure the odds of becoming pregnant in any given month. A fertile woman in her 20's has a 20% chance of conceiving every month. When this woman is 30, her monthly probability is about 10% to 15%. In her late 30's, it's perhaps 8%. These odds don't change with succeeding months of nonpregnancy.

Whether any given couple will achieve pregnancy, and when, remains something of a mystery. My example isn't atypical. Fertility treatments begun on my 36th birthday produced a baby before my 37th. The same treatments at 37-plus produced no results, so after six months I stopped them. Two years and no further treatments later, I found myself unexpectedly pregnant.

This sort of phenomenon was reported on in *The New England Journal of Medicine* in November 1983. A total of 1145 couples were diagnosed as infertile; of 597 treated for infertility, 41% became pregnant, and of 548 not treated, 35% became pregnant. Of the pregnancies in treated couples, 31% occurred either 3 months after medical treatment had stopped or 12 months after surgery and so were considered treatment-independent conceptions. The researchers concluded that there is a high potential for spontaneous cure of infertility.

So when do you start to worry? At what point do you have a problem? A cautious recommendation is to see a doctor if you're 32 or 33 and haven't become pregnant within six months. Other experts feel that six months is too short a span—it doesn't allow sufficient time for the mathematical probabilities to work themselves out. Therefore, a year is often suggested as the appropriate time span. If you're becoming upset about not conceiving, that may be the time to seek medical help, and this will obviously vary from couple to couple. A man and woman in their late 20's or very early 30's may feel no pressure if years elapse with no pregnancy. A couple in their mid or late 30's will react quite differently.

Failure to achieve pregnancy that has lasted long enough to be perceived by a couple as infertility creates a great deal of stress and tension, both for the individuals alone and within the marital relationship. Most people assume that when they want to become pregnant, they will; an inability to reproduce strikes deep at a person's self-image. Anxiety levels soar; a sense of loss and inadequacy grows, fed by the questions (discreet or blunt) of presumably well-meaning friends and relatives. Husband and wife begin to look at each other with suspicion and unease; each may seek to transfer his or her guilt feelings to the other. Awareness of childlessness becomes acute; a frustrated potential mother jealously notices pregnant women and other people's babies. This happened to several of the mothers I interviewed who had gone through a period of infertility. Irene recalled scanning every restaurant she entered and counting the pregnant women. Connie at 36 was wrenched by jealousy when her 35-year-old sister gave birth.

Optimum sexual relations, which are so necessary now, become increasingly difficult to maintain, especially when performance on schedule is required. The scheduling itself can be stressful, so sex is experienced as a staged production rather than an expression of affection and pleasure. The schedule— say, every 48 hours, no more and no less—may be interpreted as deprivation or overwork.

Mood swings are not uncommon. Mine were fairly typical while taking fertility treatments. I steeled myself against becoming ecstatic when a period was overdue and felt enormously depressed when I found I was not pregnant. I railed at the fates for this perceived cruelty—allowing me to think I might be pregnant and then letting me down terribly. When you want a baby very badly, you can know it is irrational to have these highs and lows and yet rationally not be able to prevent their occurrence.

You should keep two things in mind when dealing with these psychological difficulties. First, neither virility/maleness nor femininity/femaleness is equivalent to fertility. A man is virile whether his ejaculate produces children or not. A woman is a complete female whether she carries a baby or not. Second, a failure to conceive is almost always caused by a combination of male–female factors. A woman with somewhat irregular ovulation might remain nonpregnant if her husband has a relatively low or poor sperm count, whereas she might conceive with little delay if her husband has an abundance of vigorous sperm. Placing blame on one partner or the other is meaningless and counterproductive.

Once you've decided to seek medical help for a failure to conceive, to whom do you turn? Find a specialist. An experienced gynecologist can identify many female reproductive problems; just be sure he or she is in fact an expert in fertility matters. Or your gynecologist may refer you to a doctor who specializes in fertility treatment. Your male partner may also be sent to a urologist; be sure, however, that the urologist is experienced in fertility diagnosis and treatment—many are not. Your family practitioner could be the first person to consult; he or she can make an initial assessment, guide you to a specialist, and provide some essential psychological support.

Treatment of infertility will vary from doctor to doctor. You should know whether your regimen is well established or experimental. Once you've selected your doctor, however, stick with her or him long enough to give the course of treatment a chance to be effective. This can be a real problem if you're moving frequently during this period. Treatment could take time, especially since age-related factors may have combined with other causes of lowered fertility. It may not take long, though. As many as 20% of "infertile" couples who consult a doctor for the condition find themselves pregnant before undertaking any treatment other than an initial examination!

Some of the frustrations of dealing with fertility problems are exemplified by Beth's experience. (The procedures mentioned here are described in detail later in this chapter.) She decided to become pregnant eight months after her marriage at 35. When six months elapsed with no conception, Beth consulted a specialist; for the next six months, Beth monitored her basal body temperature daily. Since Beth was still not pregnant, her husband, Bill, had a sperm count done. Beth herself underwent a series of tests, including a endometrial biopsy, air insufflation of the fallopian tubes, and four examinations of cervical mucus. These procedures and the accompanying office visits were both time-consuming and expensive. Costs rose to $800, and Beth's health-insurance company balked at paying for fertility investigation as opposed to "nonelective" gynecological treatments. Beth discontinued the testing when she was laid off from her job; unemployed, she worries that she and Bill now can't afford a child for a year or two while she also remains anxious about her ability to conceive.

The Physiology of Conception

Before understanding the causes of and treatments for infertility, you need to have the normal conception process clearly in mind. The vagina is the elastic canal into which sperm is ejaculated. The cervix is the entrance to the uterus, or womb; the opening is protected by a thick mucus, which the sperm must penetrate in order to enter the uterus. Once past the cervical mucus, which becomes thin and watery during ovulation, sperm can remain viable for 48 hours. Only $\frac{1}{10}$ of 1% of the sperm in an ejaculate will make it this far; but since 200 million sperm may have been initially deposited, that tiny fraction can amount to 200,000 potential fertilizers. These so-far successful sperm move through the uterus to the fallopian tubes, some right away, some after a period of time. They then enter the tubes, again not all at once but in controlled numbers. Perhaps only 200 to 400 of the original 200 million sperm actually enter a tube. Even fewer are likely to get near an egg. If one of these sperm does encounter a recently ovulated egg halfway up the tube, fertilization occurs. Interestingly, it is only after sperm have been outside the male for some time, probably several hours, that they become capable of fertilization, a process called capacitation.

The fallopian tubes, attached to the top of the uterus at opposite sides, are two extremely narrow canals that each widen at the end into a flower- or trumpet-like opening called the fimbria. Gabriele Fallopius, their 16th-century discoverer, christened the tubes "trumpets of the uterus." Each fimbria hovers over one of the two ovaries, each of which is connected not to the tubes but to the uterus by a stalk-like ligament. Within the walnut-sized ovaries are the hundreds of thousands of immature eggs, or oocytes, you were born with.

Approximately once a month, stimulated by interacting hormones, an egg matures and erupts through the surface of its ovary. The ovaries don't take turns extruding eggs each month; it's a random pattern, sometimes one, sometimes the other. If one ovary ceases to function entirely, the other can produce a monthly egg. The waiting fimbria draws the egg out of the abdominal cavity into the fallopian tube. Tiny hairs called cilia move the egg along the tube until it is halfway to the uterus. It is here that fertilization must take place, and within 24 hours after the egg left the ovary. Only one sperm can penetrate, after which the egg completely seals itself off from all other sperm.

After fertilization, the egg divides and redivides in the tube. After several days, the embryo passes on down the tube to the uterus, where it implants in the uterine lining and begins to develop rapidly. A particular hormone is produced only after successful implantation, which is technically called "nidation," from the French word *nid*, "nest." It's the presence of this hormone that results in a positive pregnancy test.

Production of sperm is accomplished in the testicles, or testes, which are enclosed in the scrotum, also called the scrotal sac. The scrotum is located outside the body because normal body temperature is too high for sperm production, which requires a constant temperature of 94°F. The testicles produce both the male hormone, testosterone, and sperm. The hormone is manufactured in cells within the testicles and absorbed into the body by tiny veins. The sperm is made in hundreds of delicate tubules and carried through an incredibly tiny, convoluted, and long tube called the epididymis from the testicles to the vas deferens. While journeying through the epididymis—it takes a little less than two weeks—the sperm develop their ability to swim vigorously and straight ahead, a key requirement for fertilization. The epididymis empties the sperm into the vas deferens, the sperm duct. During intercourse, the sperm move through the vas deferens to the ejaculatory duct and into the urethra, which is inside the penis. At orgasm, the sperm is ejaculated out of the urethra, pushed on by fluid from the seminal vesicles and prostate gland.

Notice from this description that production of the male hormone and its absorption into the body are completely separate from production and ejaculation of sperm. Also, most of the ejaculate consists of seminal fluid, not sperm. In other words, a man's "maleness" and ability to ejaculate have nothing to do with sperm production or fertility and are unaffected by vasectomy (severing of the vas deferens).

Diagnosing and Treating Infertility

In almost all cases, the reason for infertility can be found even if it can't be corrected. First, of course, a thorough diagnosis must be made, which can take three months or more and involve three or four office visits (more for the wife, less for the husband). Before even seeing you initially, your doctor may ask you to record your basal body temperature every day for three to six months to get a picture of your ovulatory pattern.

Both you and your partner should go to the first office visit, during which your doctor will discuss infertility and its causes and will take a complete medical history of both of you. It is extremely important that you be as accurate and honest as possible. You should remember past illnesses, infections, and surgery, thoroughly report your menstrual and reproductive history, and accurately describe your current marital and sexual relationship. A drug history of both you and your partner is also very important. All of these factors affect fertility. My fertility specialist spent an hour and a half at the first visit getting this very detailed history.

One of the next steps is simple sperm testing, since it is quite easy to evaluate the man's sperm and more difficult and involved to evaluate the woman's role in infertility (although usually easier to treat). A sperm count and/or a postcoital test is taken. You will be told to refrain from intercourse for a few days to be sure the sperm level is not depleted; then you must collect a semen sample and, keeping it at the appropriate temperature, bring it in within two hours for testing. Because most of the sperm is in the first portion of the ejaculate, it is important to collect all of it, best done by masturbation, in a wide-mouthed jar. Also, because sperm counts vary widely from sample to sample, at least two samples should be analyzed.

A sperm count reveals more than just the number of sperm. Of greatest importance is the concentration of sperm—how many there are per cubic centimeter—and their motility—the rate and quality of their movement. Also checked is sperm morphology, or structure. Abnormally shaped sperm are incapable of fertilization, so it is a poor indication for fertility if a semen sample contains very large numbers of such sperm. However, there is no agreement about what a normal or adequate sperm count is. You will have to discuss the results thoroughly with your physician in order to make a sound evaluation.

A second sperm test is the postcoital test, in which a sample of your cervical mucus after intercourse is tested. Fertilization can't take place if the sperm can't penetrate the mucus;

this test checks for the presence of active, vigorous sperm in the sample. It also indicates if sufficient sperm are present. Timing is critical, though, because the cervical mucus only permits penetration by sperm during a short time each month, and only if the sample is taken just then will the postcoital test be valid. While the test must be done reasonably soon after intercourse, you don't need, literally, to run from the bedroom to the doctor's office, zipping your fly and buttoning your blouse; just get there for testing within 24 hours.

Unfortunately, although sperm testing is the simplest and most important initial procedure in infertility screening, it is vigorously resisted by those men who continue to associate virility and potency with fertility. The concept of a sperm count is overwhelmingly threatening to their masculinity. A thorough explanation of the physiology involved may change such a man's mind. Otherwise, the wife will have to go through a series of time-consuming and costly tests that may give inconclusive results if the husband's role cannot be evaluated. Refusal to allow a sperm count is also an automatic assignation of blame to the woman. "It can't be my fault—so it must be yours." This exacerbates a situation already fraught with stress.

Even if a man's sperm count shows abnormalities, his wife can easily be a contributing factor to their infertility. Physical exams of both husband and wife can reveal relatively simple or easily diagnosable problems such as, for the husband; varicose veins in the testicles, or, for the wife, benign tumors or cysts. Lab studies for both partners can check factors such as hormone levels and infections.

Causes Common to Men and Women

Several conditions can affect fertility in both male and female. The most obvious but, strangely, most often overlooked factor is the level and type of sexual activity. Some couples do not become pregnant because they simply don't have intercourse often. Once or twice a month is not enough! Long periods of abstinence reduce the number of fresh, vigorous sperm in the semen. On the other hand, daily ejaculation reduces sperm count, which may have an adverse effect for a man of borderline fertility. Optimal frequency of intercourse for conception is about once every two days. Infrequent or irregular intercourse can easily miss the short period of about 48 hours each month when conception can take place. Or the pattern of a couple's life may cause the time of fertility to fall consistently into a noncoital period—for instance, if either partner goes away on a regular business trip just then. Also, certain sexual positions and techniques favor conception by reducing sperm leakage from the vagina, such as the time-honored missionary position and having the woman remain in bed with feet slightly elevated after intercourse. Douching—which most doctors warn against in any case—can wash away sperm. Solving problems in this area is a simple matter of adjusting timing, frequency, and method of intercourse and can be particularly important in cases of marginal fertility.

Sexual dysfunction naturally affects the ability to conceive. Couples have a tendency to shrink from discussing this, but there is no point in going through an extensive fertility evalua-tion if no sperm is reaching the cervix in the first place. Women's problems in this area include painful intercourse, dislike of sex, and vaginismus, an extreme tightening of the vaginal muscles. Inadequate lubrication may cause or aggravate the problem. Psychological factors can also inhibit ovulation. Male problems include impotence, premature ejaculation, and retarded ejaculation, all of which mean sperm is not deposited in the vagina. Sexual dysfunction is not necessarily psychologi-cal in origin. Screening for physiological causes should come first. Sixty percent of male impotence can now be traced to medical problems, including endocrine imbalances, vascular insufficiency, and the effect of drugs. Diabetes, for example, can cause retrograde ejaculation—the sperm is expelled into the bladder—a condition that can usually be easily corrected. If no physical causes of dysfunction are found, counseling can have very successful results.

Another common group of factors affecting fertility—also sometimes overlooked—is what can be called system disor-ders: poor nutrition (including under- and over-weight), infec-tion, chronic disease and its treatment, stress, fatigue. Nutri-tional levels can, for example, affect ovulation, as can extremely strenuous physical activity such as marathon running, which can completely suppress ovulation. Sperm production can be temporarily depressed by infections, by various drugs taken to treat a temporary infection or by chronic disease, and by high fever or another source of excess heat. Too-high scrotal temperatures can be induced by hot tubs, saunas, fashionably tight pants, or even driving long distances. Stress and fatigue can impair sexual performance and alter ovulatory patterns. You and your doctor should screen carefully for the presence of any of these difficulties and act to correct them.

Infection, current and past, can have a profound effect on fertility. The most serious consequence of infection is scarring and adhesions, which remain long after the infection itself has cleared up. Scar tissue is especially likely to cause blockages of the very delicate fallopian tubes and the epididymis. Certain infections can affect the reproductive system; particularly devastating are venereal and pelvic inflammatory disease. The older you are, the more likely you are to have had one of these, especially if you have been sexually active with a number of different partners. Venereal disease is epidemic now; both chlamydia and gonorrhea are common causes of infertility. Chlamydia affects more than three million people a year in the United States; it comes in several disease forms and is very difficult to diagnose. Its symptoms resemble those of several other infections. They may not be apparent and they may be disguised because another disease, such as gonorrhea, is also present. One of the major diseases caused by chlamydia organisms is genital tract infection, resulting in inflammation of the testes in men and of the fallopian tubes (plus the cervix and uterus) in women—both potential threats to fertility if left untreated. Antibiotics will cure a chlamydial infection, once a diagnosis is made. Another genital tract infection called T mycoplasma probably also plays an important role in infertility, according to the *New England Journal of Medicine* (March 3, 1983); when T mycoplasma is eradicated, 60% of affected, previously infertile couples achieve successful pregnancy.

IUD users are twice as likely as nonusers to suffer from pelvic inflammatory disease and therefore tubal defects and uterine scarring. Some authorities even suggest you not use an IUD until after you've had all the children you plan to have. Common vaginal yeast infections do not appear to affect future fertility, although they do need treatment.

There is some indication that long-term, steady use of marijuana affects fertility in both men and women. Steady male users have been found to have changed hormone levels, lowered sperm counts, and more abnormal sperm, while steady female users have experienced changes in ovulation. Alcohol, too, can depress sperm count and movement; it can also adversely affect sexual performance. Changes induced by marijuana and alcohol may present no problem when you're in your 20's and very fertile, but they could be significant when your fertility begins to decline in your 30's.

Causes of Male Infertility

Certain possible causes of male infertility are easily diagnosed and treated, but many are not. Most common is a varicocele—a varicose vein of the testicle, which is almost always found on the left side and usually develops during puberty. The enlarged veins allow blood to pool in the testes, raising scrotal temperature. A varicocele does affect sperm production, but it does not produce infertility in all men. In fact, 10% to 15% of normally fertile men have a varicocele. For infertile men, though, surgery called varicolectomy to correct the condition is the most successful of all fertility treatments. In 75% of cases the sperm count is improved, and pregnancy subsequently results in up to 50% of cases. Another procedure, recently approved by the FDA, is insertion of a tiny device into the varicose vein to prevent pooling of blood; this form of varicocele treatment can be done on an outpatient basis.

Some male children have undescended testicles; if this condition isn't corrected by age one, the high body temperature will permanently affect sperm-producing ability. A man with only one testicle, though, is quite capable of fathering a child. Adult mumps are rare, but can affect the testicles and severely reduce sperm count; mumps vaccine, now available, should be taken advantage of. Any sudden scrotal swelling needs immediate diagnosis to prevent permanent blockage or damage. Testicle injury can hinder sperm production and free passage of sperm through the tubes.

Because the sperm must pass through so much intricate tubing—especially the epididymis—blockages are another fairly common cause of male infertility. The obstruction may have existed since birth or it may have developed after an infection created scar tissue. Previous surgery may also have injured part of the system, especially the vas deferens. Surgery to correct these conditions has always been very difficult because of the delicate nature of the tubing. However, modern microsurgery is rapidly improving results.

Hormone levels are also critical to a man's fertility. However, treatment to correct imbalances is the least successful approach to curing infertility. Hormone therapy for men is still essentially experimental, as are dietary regimens.

Causes of Female Infertility

Although 40% to 50% of fertility problems involve male factors, many cannot be treated successfully. Fortunately, correction of the female factor(s) alone can often produce pregnancy.

A woman's medical history can be very revealing, showing nonnormal ovulation or disclosing incidents that could have affected reproductive organs, such as induced abortions, miscarriage, surgery, childbirth accompanied by severe bleeding, ectopic pregnancies, and infections and illnesses. Prior abortions using the vacuum method rather than dilation and curettage (D & C) do not, however, affect subsequent ability to conceive, as was once believed, although the old D & C method may have negative consequences. Researchers reporting this conclusion in the February 1984 issue of *Obstetrics and Gynecology* found that women who had three or more induced abortions actually had a higher pregnancy rate after the abortions than other women.

A pelvic exam can reveal structural abnormalities, tumors, or cysts. Tubal blockage can be diagnosed by X-ray and dye (a procedure with the side effect of temporarily boosting fertility), by passing gas or saline solution through the tubes, or by direct observation via tiny lighted telescopes. These procedures are not so much painful as uncomfortable; the dye material can be quite messy for a while afterward.

To discover whether you ovulate regularly or irregularly, you must check your ovulatory pattern. The best way to do this is to record your basal body temperature (BBT) daily; this can only be done accurately *before* you stir from bed in the morning. Specially marked, easy-to-read thermometers are available for this, along with recording charts, at any drug store. After ovulation, your body temperature rises one degree. The day *before* this rise is the day you ovulate. Some women experience a drop in temperature one day before the rise. The temperature drops again when menstruation begins. By recording your BBT every day for several months you will get a good picture of your ovulatory cycle. Because the temperature changes are caused by hormones, the BBT chart shows whether your hormone production occurs on schedule. The chart also indicates whether or not you ovulate and on what schedule. Once you know the schedule, you can figure out pretty accurately when your fertile period is—about 14 days *before* your next period begins—and time intercourse accordingly. Remember, though, that you are no longer fertile once the temperature has risen; you must have intercourse a day or two before the rise in order for vigorous sperm to be present just after ovulation.

While you're keeping track of your BBT, your doctor may also check your cervical mucus at intervals during your cycle. Pregnancy cannot occur unless the cervix opens and the mucus changes consistency to permit passage of sperm. This only happens, and at the right time in mid-cycle, with proper hormone stimulation. A cervical exam will indicate if this phase of your cycle is normal. Vaginal pH, too, can be tested. The postcoital study already mentioned shows if the sperm are in fact successfully penetrating the cervical mucus. If not, the problem might be sperm motility, which could be improved by a higher sperm count, or it might be a lack of estrogen, which could be remedied by hormone treatment. Cervicitis—cervical infection, often noxious to sperm—can also be diagnosed and treated. Much less commonly found, but sometimes misdiagnosed as present, are actual sperm antibodies, which may be controlled by use of a condom for a period of time. After a period of non-exposure to sperm, the mucus will presumably no longer contain sperm antibodies. Resumption of non-condom intercourse can now hopefully result in impregnation.

Another examination of the ovulatory cycle is an endometrial biopsy. A bit of the uterine lining is removed and studied for normal development at the right time during the cycle. This can reveal any inflammation of the lining that needs clearing up. Again, it is an uncomfortable but not really painful procedure.

Common treatment of female infertility involves either drug therapy to induce or maintain ovulation or surgery to correct growths and adhesions. We've all heard of fertility drugs. Their primary purpose is to induce regular ovulation, the lack of which is a major cause of female infertility. They are successful in accomplishing that goal 80% of the time. However, fertility drugs are expensive. Clomid, one of the most widely used, costs about $4.25 per tablet; 5, 10, or even 20 tablets per month may be prescribed, so a six-month course of treatment can set you back as much as $570 for the drug alone. Another, more powerful, drug is Pergonal, administered by injection for 9 to 12 days. You have to pay for the drug and possibly the daily office visits to receive it.

Ironically, Clomid was originally studied as a contraceptive, but was found, instead, to stimulate ovulation. The problem is that fertility drugs can overstimulate the ovaries and thus cause multiple births. The probabilities depend on what drug is being used. For Clomid, the multiple-birth rate is 7% to 10%, while for Pergonal it's 20%; the national average for all multiple births is 1%. When I took fertility treatments and found myself pregnant for the first time, I braced myself for a litter; I was worried about the children dying at birth or being handicapped, and about my inability emotionally and financially to mother a group. I must admit I was relieved when ultrasound showed just one developing fetus. Of course, the odds heavily favored a single pregnancy.

One use of drug therapy is of particular interest to the over-35 woman. It can restimulate ovulation after discontinuation of the Pill if regular menstrual function has not returned unassisted. If you're in your mid 30's, you may have been on the Pill for 10 or 15 years or more; your ovaries have been stopped in their tracks all that time. They may not snap back into working order when you go off the Pill, a condition called "post-Pill amenorrhea." The problem is particularly likely to occur if you had irregular menstrual periods before you began taking the Pill. In fact, irregular menstrual cycles may be an indication not to start using the Pill until after you've finished your childbearing.

You may not have heard of endometriosis. Many people haven't, yet in women of childbearing age, it is probably more common than appendicitis and is a culprit in 20% to 40% of female infertility cases. The endometrium is the lining of the uterus. Bits of it can detach, enter the pelvic cavity, and attach to whatever is there, especially the tubes and ovaries. During menstruation, this tissue bleeds, then heals; eventually scars and adhesions grow. Because the uterine cells probably migrate during menstruation, the more menstrual cycles you go through, the more likely you are to develop endometriosis. In other words, the older you are, the more likely you are to be affected by this major cause of infertility. Extremely painful periods are a possible symptom of the condition. The best treatment is pregnancy, which usually destroys the growth; therefore, hormones to simulate pregnancy can be taken as a cure. The subsequent pregnancy rate is 50%. Surgery can also remove the scar tissue. Even untreated, many women with endometriosis will, in time, eventually become pregnant.

Other surgical treatments of infertility involve corrections of malformations and removal of tumors and other growths from the reproductive organs. A closed cervix can be surgically opened, and an incompetent cervix—one that opens much too soon during pregnancy—can in many cases be successfully sutured long enough to sustain a pregnancy. Fibroid tumors, often found on the uterus, may interfere with pregnancy, depending on where they're located. A small one may be no problem, but fibroid tumors tend to grow. For this reason, if you have one, it's probably best to proceed right away with whatever pregnancies you plan to have. Surgery can remove the growth, but scarring may still prevent successful pregnancy.

Perhaps the most common use of fertility-related surgery is to correct blocked fallopian tubes. Tubal problems are involved in about 20% of infertility. The opening along which the egg travels is tiny, and the tubular muscles must remain flexible. Neither egg nor sperm will move along the tube unless propelled by the cilia which, once damaged, are unlikely to heal. Any sort of infection—one you may not even remember—can cause permanent scarring of the tubes. So can endometriosis, abdominal surgery, and tubal pregnancy. Surgical success depends on the nature and location of the blockage; internal scarring of the tubes is much more difficult to correct than external scarring. As with blockage of the male tubes, microsurgery is improving the success ratio of this treatment. However, tubal surgery somewhat increases the risk of a subsequent tubal pregnancy.

Elective vasectomy and tubal ligation are permanent methods of birth control, in which, respectively, the vas deferens and the fallopian tubes are severed. Ironically, as the divorce and remarriage rates climb, increasing numbers of men and women are going to their doctors saying, "I had my tubes tied; I've remarried; I want another child. What can you do for me?" They are seeking to reverse these presumably irreversible procedures. Microsurgery does make it possible sometimes. Vasectomy can be reversed, but it is a very intricate and delicate procedure. Tubal resection is similarly possible; success can depend on how much of the tube was destroyed originally—damage can be extensive.

Innovative Options

What if, despite everyone's best efforts, you still cannot conceive? The answer used to be adoption. Because of the scarcity of normal healthy infants, that's no longer much of an option. Birth control, abortion, and single parenthood have effectively dried up the supply of adoptable infants. Because so few are available, you're likely to be rejected by an agency as too old if you're over 35. Adoption is, of course, still possible, but it may take as long as or longer than attempts to treat infertility, with no guarantee of success.

Private adoption is becoming more common because it avoids some of these problems. You won't be summarily refused because of age, and you won't be placed at the bottom of a long waiting list. However, private adoption can be difficult to arrange. You need an attorney, because the legal procedure for such an adoption varies from state to state, with some states outlawing it entirely. Friends of mine had to move from Connecticut to Florida in order to adopt a child privately. It can be expensive too. While you can not pay for the baby, you will in most cases pay the medical and legal costs and may in some states pay the pregnant woman's prenatal living expenses as well. Private adoption is often arranged by an attorney acting as a sort of adoption agent, whom you can be directed to by a fertility specialist, friends, or acquaintances.

Today's solution to childlessness is more likely to be artificial insemination, whereby sperm is mechanically introduced into the cervical canal. This comes in two variations—AID (with donor sperm) and AIH (with homologous, or the husband's, sperm). AIH is not usually any more successful than intercourse, but it can be tried when the husband has a low sperm count (using the portion of the ejaculate with the greatest concentration of vigorous sperm) or is unable to ejaculate in his wife's vagina.

The vast majority of cases use AID. Consent forms are necessary and the legitimacy of the child depends on state law. The child may be legitimate only if the proper forms are signed by husband and wife, only if the insemination was performed by a licensed physician, or only if the insemination followed prescribed procedures. Most state laws are moot on the AID child's legitimacy; a few of these nevertheless require the husband to support such a child. Single women and gay couples may request AID; the response is up to the individual doctor.

Estimates of the number of AID babies born annually are hard to come by. It's a topic not openly discussed, because of a couple's reluctance to admit that a husband has been unable to impregnate his wife, while a stranger's sperm has succeeded. Donors are most often medical students or interns. The donor's and the husband's characteristics are carefully matched, even for athletic abilities. The same donor can be used a second time so the children's inherited characteristics will be the same.

The success rate for AID is quite high; up to 80% of AID subjects become pregnant in the first year. As in natural insemination, however, maternal age affects the likelihood of conception. This was made clear by the results of 404 courses of treatment by AID. The older a woman was, the more monthly cycles of insemination were required to achieve pregnancy, and the less chance she had of conceiving at all. A chart showing this follows.

In vitro fertilization—"test-tube pregnancy"—is now being performed regularly and with success, but it is a complex procedure and not at all widespread. It involves aspiration of an ovulated egg, introduction of sperm to the egg in a tissue-culture medium—the "test tube"—and placement of the resulting embryo in the mother's uterus, prepared for pregnancy by hormone stimulation.

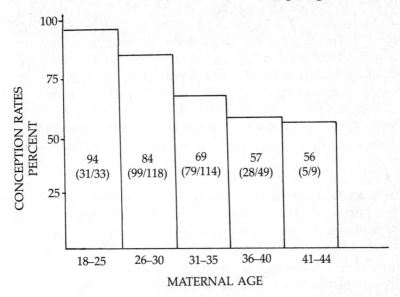

Conception rates with AID within one year versus maternal age. (Figures in parentheses indicate number of conceptions and number of cases.)

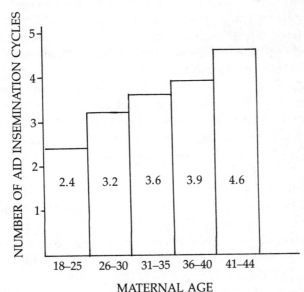

Number of cycles of artificial insemination with donor sperm required to conceive versus maternal age.

[Source: Michael R. Virro, M.D., et al., "Pregnancy Outcome in 242 Conceptions after Artificial Insemination with Donor Sperm and Effects of Maternal Age on the Prognosis for Successful Pregnancy," reprinted with permission of the *American Journal of Obstetrics and Gynecology*, 148:5 (March 1, 1984), p. 521–22.]

The success ratio of single implantation is not high. To boost it, multiple embryos may be injected into the uterus, which then raises the risk of multiple pregnancy. The overall chance of success is only 20% per attempt according to *Science* magazine (Sept. 16, 1983) or 30% according to *Lancet,* the British medical journal (Dec. 3, 1983). Maternal age affects the outcome; *Lancet* reports that women 35 to 39 are twice as likely to abort a test-tube pregnancy as women 25 to 29. Each attempt costs an average of $3000 to $4000 in the United States, although some centers charge more.

In vitro fertilization recently resulted in a bizarre situation that attracted international attention. In 1981, Mario and Elsa Rios of Los Angeles traveled to a leading clinic in the state of Victoria, Australia, where several eggs were aspirated from Mrs. Rios, inseminated by donor sperm, and frozen. The Rioses, however, were killed in a plane crash in 1983 before the embryos could be implanted in Mrs. Rios. The couple left no instructions about the orphan embryos. A son of Mr. Rios by a former marriage moved to bar the embryos from a share in his father's substantial estate. With attention thus focused on the frozen orphans, the clinic announced its plans to destroy them. Women from around the world clamored to adopt and be implanted with the embryos. Much public debate ensued, with Victoria's state law being amended to permit adoption of orphaned embryos. The clinic recently agreed to thaw and implant, although the embryos are not expected to survive because freezing techniques were not so well developed in 1981 as they are today. Other state governments in Australia and the United States are now debating legislation to cover such situations.

In spite of legal complexities and expense, use of this method of conception will spread as increasing numbers of medical centers offer it. The American Fertility Society maintains a continually updated list of such centers; to obtain a copy, write to the Society at 2131 Magnolia Avenue, Suite 20, Birmingham, Alabama 35256.

A sideline of all this study of conception is the possibility of sex preselection—choosing or influencing the sex of your child. Sex is determined at the moment of conception, depending on whether the fertilizing sperm contains an X (girl) or Y (boy) chromosome. Various researchers have reported differences between X and Y sperm. According to one theory, the Y sperm swim faster, so if you want a boy, you should have intercourse right at ovulation—the Y's will beat the X's to the egg. If, however, you want a girl, have intercourse a few days before ovulation; the X sperm live longer and will still be around to fertilize the egg after the Y sperm have expired.

Another theory is that X sperm tolerate acid conditions better than Y sperm, so you should time intercourse to hit your peak alkalinity (just as you ovulate and/or just after an alkaline douche) to boost your chances of conceiving a boy. Conversely, intercourse a day or two before ovulation and just after an acid douche should favor conception of a girl.

Results are *not* guaranteed; there's plenty of contradictory evidence. And feminists take note. Studies show that people prefer males for their first-born. If sex preselection works and if people continue this preference, we'll have fewer girls with the purported first-born characteristics of high achievement and leadership.

In summing up, it's a lot easier to avoid infertility, if possible, than to treat it. How can you do this? First, try to avoid foreseeable health problems. If you're planning to have children in the future, stay fit, keep healthy by maintaining good nutrition, and get prompt treatment for any infections or abnormalities. You don't always know that a problem is developing, but be alert to possible symptoms and discuss them with your doctor. Second, try to estimate your and your mate's fertility *now* even if you don't plan a pregnancy until some time in the future. Review your medical history, monitor your ovulatory pattern, have a medical checkup. Then, if a problem seems to exist, treatment, if indicated, can begin now so you will be less likely to experience fertility problems in your late 30's when they could be critical. Finally, if possible, plan at what age you want your last child, not your first. Don't wait till you're 34 to try to conceive if you want to finish multiple childbearing by the time you're 37. Either start sooner or revise your age limit.

The treatment of fertility problems is vastly more advanced today than it used to be. New techniques like microsurgery and in vitro fertilization promise further advances. If you do have trouble conceiving, the chances that your difficulty can be overcome are very high.

CHAPTER 3

THE FIRST TRIMESTER OF PREGNANCY

It's probably happened at least once to all of us: Your period is overdue, maybe only by a few days; inevitably, the thought forms—am I pregnant?

If you haven't been trying to conceive, you'll chide yourself for overreacting and you'll attempt to dismiss the possibility for now. But for each day that goes by without the onset of menstruation, the thought continues to nag at you, and you experience half-stifled feelings of hope, fear, anticipation, anxiety.

If you have been trying to become pregnant, you most likely have been watching and studying your menstrual cycles in an intensely focused way. As soon as your period is a day or two late you may start evaluating every nuance of your body, seeking signs of pregnancy. You'll try to temper your feelings of joy and anticipation, for fear of a tremendous letdown in the event the overdue period should finally arrive.

If menstruation continues not to occur, you'll seek confirmation of your pregnancy or nonpregnancy. Avoid the tendency of some over-35 women to dismiss the possibility of having conceived—"I'm too old to be pregnant!" "I've never gotten pregnant before [or not for the past 10 years], so I can't be pregnant now!" A sensitive blood test called Beta HCG can tell you if you're pregnant within 48 hours of conception, long before your period is due. This test is generally used only by women who are either very anxious to be pregnant or very anxious not to be, and then only when the period is a few days late. The more common pregnancy test checks the urine for the presence of HCG, a hormone produced only during pregnancy.

You can buy a home test kit at any drug store or have a test performed by your doctor. Levels of HCG in the urine may not be high enough to give a clear positive result until six weeks after your last period. A test done sooner can give a false negative.

By the time your period is two weeks late, however, you're one month pregnant, since conception will have occurred approximately two weeks after the onset of your last period. A pregnancy test may only confirm what you already know. There are some very early symptoms of pregnancy, mostly triggered by increased hormone levels, which begin to climb within days of conception. Your breasts may feel tender and full. Your lower abdomen may feel congested and you might have some cramping. You will probably miss your period, although slight bleeding or spotting isn't uncommon. You might find yourself urinating more frequently. You may feel nauseous, especially in the morning, and terribly tired by late afternoon or early evening. You may also simply "feel" pregnant—many women report a sense of being pregnant that is a purely subjective phenomenon, independent of any medical test or physical symptoms. I had such a strong sense of being pregnant, I disbelieved the negative results of my Beta HCG test and insisted on a urinalysis. The positive result confirmed my feeling; the laboratory, it turned out, had read the wrong line on the computer screen when reporting a negative outcome for the first test.

When you think you may be pregnant, monitor yourself for these early warning symptoms. Once your period is several weeks overdue, consult a doctor to confirm the pregnancy. Early diagnosis is important so you can begin prenatal care promptly or decide on an abortion earlier rather than later. Deciding to terminate a pregnancy can be terribly difficult, especially if you are ambivalent or if your partner strongly favors a different decision than yours. It's also particularly hard if you already have children, and can contemplate the graphic evidence of what a pregnancy grows into. My friend Cindy, whose daughter was a nursery school classmate of my son, was deeply troubled when she found herself unexpectedly pregnant at the age of 40. Despite the enthusiasm of her husband Jack, an established engineer, who urged her to go ahead with the pregnancy, Cindy felt her preexisting parental responsibilities were a strong motivation for terminating the pregnancy. She, like many other older women faced with an unplanned pregnancy, seriously considered abortion. Her decision took time, and early confirmation of pregnancy gave her that time.

A pregnancy book is not complete without a detailed discussion of developments during the nine months of gestation. This chapter and the two following, therefore, describe the three trimesters of pregnancy. While much of this is not age specific, attention is drawn to aspects of particular interest to the over-35 woman and her partner.

Fetal Development in the First Three Months

You may not look pregnant, and you may not feel pregnant, but your baby has been developing at an astonishing rate ever since conception. On the journey from the fallopian tube to the uterus, the cells of the newly fertilized egg divide and redivide many times. When the ovum reaches the uterus, it embeds itself in the uterine wall. (Some women experience slight bleeding at implantation—about a week before the period is due—another early symptom of pregnancy.) Now called an embryo, the baby needs nutrients to sustain its rapid growth. Finger- or root-like projections called villi reach deep into the uterine lining until they are surrounded by the mother's blood vessels. This is the beginning of the placenta, through which oxygen, nutrients, and wastes are exchanged. Maternal and fetal blood do not actually mix; the substances are transferred through the thin walls of the villi.

The next several months are critical to the developing baby. All of the major organs and structures are formed; they continue to grow and develop throughout pregnancy, but it is in the first trimester—the first three months after conception—that cells differentiate and produce a fully formed potential human being.

At six weeks after your last period, the embryo (now one month old) is about ¼-inch long. It has a large head and small tail, rather like a tadpole, and the buds of arms and legs. A tiny tube that will become your baby's heart has begun to beat, and blood vessels have begun to form. The brain and spinal cord have begun to develop, as have such organs as the stomach, intestines, kidneys, and liver. Your period is now two weeks overdue, and you may just be finding out that you're pregnant—yet the developing embryo inside you already has a beating heart!

During the embryo's second month, the arms and legs grow, forming finger and toe ridges. A human face is recognizable, with primitive eyes, nose, ears, and mouth. The brain develops rapidly; other organs appear or continue to grow, including genitalia. At the end of two months, the 1½-inch-long embryo has most of its major organs and all of its body parts. It is now called a fetus.

By the end of the third month, fingers and toes are distinct and nails are forming on them. The future child's sex can be identified. The fetus moves its arms and legs, but you can't feel the movement yet. The heart is beating rapidly. The fetus can squint its eyes and open its mouth. The buds for baby teeth are in. Some of the organs have begun to function—the kidneys, for instance, are working and a little urine is secreted. After three months of growth, the one-celled, nearly invisible ovum has become a one-ounce, 3- or 4-inch-long fetus.

Changes and Common Complaints of Early Pregnancy

Small as the developing baby may be, it causes distinct changes in you—not just in your uterus, but throughout your body. Conception triggers increased production of certain hormones, especially progesterone and estrogen, which in turn stimulate the changes in your body necessary to carry through a pregnancy. Your bathroom scale may inch slowly upward in the early months, but any weight gain will be small; you won't "show" the pregnancy yet. You may welcome the earliest visible change, especially if you're normally somewhat flatchested; your breasts will swell noticeably as they grow extra fatty tissue and as blood volume increases. The dark area around your nipples will widen and darken. Before the days of pregnancy tests, these breast changes served as an early confirmation of pregnancy.

Your climbing levels of progesterone relax the involuntary muscles, allowing the uterus and the blood vessels to expand. Increased blood volume is needed to serve the needs of the growing fetus. As the uterus grows, it crowds the bladder, so you find yourself having to urinate annoyingly often. You will also breathe more rapidly, and your heart will beat faster. These physical changes have varying effects on different women in terms of how they feel during the first trimester. Some women say they never felt better than during pregnancy. Others feel good with one pregnancy and not with another. For a few women pregnancy—especially the early part—is the pits. There are a few complaints or minor ills that are not uncommon during these first three months, although you may very well not experience any of them. Fortunately, none of them except fatigue seems to be any more common for the over-35 woman than among younger mothers-to-be.

Nausea

Probably the most common complaint of early pregnancy is nausea, with or without vomiting. For some, it is a morning sickness; for others it occurs at some other particular time of day or even continues most of the day. It's caused by the high levels of pregnancy hormones, which stimulate production of stomach acids while bowel movement emptying the stomach slows down. It can make you—and your partner—regret, momentarily, that you ever got pregnant and wonder how you'll survive the next seven or eight months.

What can you do about it? Limit your intake of spicy, greasy, and fried foods and avoid any odors that trigger nausea. Get plenty of fresh air. Don't be surprised if some foods you generally love completely turn you off during pregnancy; if it repels you, don't eat it. Paradoxically, an empty stomach can aggravate the nausea, so small, frequent, bland meals can help. So can dry toast or crackers early in the morning, plus milk, juice, yogurt, or cottage cheese just before going to bed. Some women find carbonated beverages easy to get down, but in general, it's been found best not to drink liquids with meals. Fruits, fruit juices, and high-protein foods keep your blood-sugar levels high; low levels can prompt nausea. If the condition is so bad you cannot keep anything down, even liquids, you need to call your practitioner. Medication can be prescribed, although it is best to avoid medications whenever possible, especially during this first trimester. The most effective cure for this nausea is time: it usually disappears by the 12th week.

Fatigue

Fatigue, another frequently experienced and annoying complaint of early pregnancy, can be induced by progesterone, a hormone produced abundantly during pregnancy. You'll find yourself yawning in mid afternoon and barely able to keep your eyes open after dinner. One well-traveled acquaintance, Patricia, spent hectic nights dining out on the Riviera the summer she was pregnant with her first child. She, her husband, and friends visited restaurants up and down the coast, setting out about 8 P.M. in keeping with the late French dinner hour. Invariably, Patricia's head hit the table before the first course was served.

Because of fatigue, you may not feel up to your normal activities during early pregnancy, especially if you are working, taking care of young children, or both. There are only two solutions: get more rest and sleep, and let time pass—you will almost certainly feel much more energetic by the end of the trimester. If you haven't much time to turn over to extra rest and sleep because of work and/or childcare, you should at least strain yourself as little as possible, let less critical tasks slide for now, and snatch a catnap whenever you can.

Constipation

Constipation, for some, proves a constant irritation throughout pregnancy. The best way to manage it is through diet. Drink lots of fluid in addition to your daily quota of milk, which can cause constipation. Dig into salads, fresh fruit, and other high-roughage foods. Add raw bran to your recipes, and try prunes and stewed fruits for dessert. Mild exercise can be helpful. Don't put off an urge to move your bowels. Stay away from laxatives and other medications; some are not safe for pregnant women.

Vaginal Discharge

Women during pregnancy normally have an increased vaginal discharge, stimulated by the pregnancy hormones. You may not consider it aesthetic, but it is completely normal and shouldn't be treated with douches, deodorants, or medications unless specifically prescribed. The iodine in many douches, for example, is absorbed by your body and can cause fetal thyroid problems. However, you don't want to contract a vaginal infection, so report any abnormal discharge—one that is bloody, yellow or green, very heavy, frothy, or foul smelling, or that burns or itches.

Remember that the baby is particularly susceptible, during early pregnancy, to a host of ills resulting from medications you might take. So stay away from them, unless they are specifically prescribed *and* the prescriber knows you are pregnant *and* you have discussed the medication with your obstetric practitioner. The effects of drugs on pregnancy are thoroughly discussed in Chapter 7.

Danger Signals

There are certain danger signals that should always be reported immediately if they occur at any time during your pregnancy. They are:

- Bleeding from the vagina, even if it is slight.
- Sudden excessive weight gain with puffiness and swelling of hands, face, or feet. Excessive weight gain is usually considered to be two pounds a week or more.
- Headache that is severe and continuous.
- Problems with your vision such as blurring, spots before your eyes, flashes of light, or dimness.
- Severe abdominal pain, either continuous or intermittent.
- Persistent or severe vomiting.
- Fever and chills.
- Sudden leakage of fluid from your vagina.
- Unusual or excessive thirst.
- Abdominal contractions before the 37th week of pregnancy occurring as often as four times in 20 minutes or eight times in an hour.

Psychological and Sexual Changes of Early Pregnancy

You can expect a lot of emotional turmoil during these nine months and beyond, and so can your partner. Your state is described as "emotional lability," which means you'll react strongly, swiftly, and unpredictably to stimuli; your moods will swing rapidly and seem extra high and extra low. When your partner remarks on instances of this behavior, you may deny it hysterically. Your vastly altered hormone levels are partly at fault. They affect your nervous system and inevitably cause some depression and/or mood confusion. Even without the hormone stimulation, you're psychologically stressed during pregnancy by identity crisis, body image alteration, and fear of the unknown. The physical and emotional states interact and interreact throughout pregnancy so that how you feel at any given time becomes a psychosomatic function.

During the first trimester, you will tend to be very introverted and self-involved, concentrating on and trying to sort out a number of new emotions and anxieties. Many women are troubled by a strong sense of ambivalence toward their newly established pregnancy. Doubts and questions abound. I'm not ready for this! How can I make myself into a mother? What's going to happen to my body? How can I take care of another child? I'm a professional person, not a pregnant woman. I'm losing my independence. Why am I doing this? I don't really want to be pregnant! This natural ambivalence causes guilt and shame, especially if the pregnancy is a wanted one. It's intensified if you are finding the first few months physically unpleasant. It's important to acknowledge the feeling as normal and common, part of coming to grips with the pregnancy.

Related to feelings of ambivalence is anxiety about the impending shift in your identity. If this is your first child, the role of mother, which you are about to assume, is unfamiliar and thus unsettling. You might have doubts about your ability to become a good or even competent parent. You'll focus on your relationship with your own mother, seeking to resolve any conflicts in your roles. As an older woman, you have an advantage here, since the resolution of parent–child conflict and establishment of a secure adult identity is usually completed by the time you're in your 30's. But while you're evolving your concepts of motherhood, you may worry about repeating patterns set by your mother. This too is common. Remember that you're free to become the type of parent you feel most comfortable being, and that everyone parents differently based on his or her own needs and reactions.

Whether it's your first or a subsequent pregnancy, you're likely to feel vulnerable and dependent, which can be very difficult to deal with if you're accustomed to feeling strong and independent. You may fear loss of the pregnancy even while you're not yet sure you even want it. This fear will be intensified if you've undergone an earlier pregnancy loss. You can fear labor and delivery, either as an unknown or as a repetition of a particularly difficult experience. You might fear the responsibility of a child, new or added. You might worry about the impact that the child will have on the relationship you've established with your partner; chances are, though, as an older couple, that you have cemented that relationship.

Most of these fears crop up during the first trimester; some will be resolved and others will continue throughout the pregnancy. Anxiety sometimes expresses itself in dreams, which may be intense and feature your baby, who may not be normal or who has been harmed, specifically by your neglect. Disturbing as these dreams are, they too are a normal part of pregnancy and not a prediction of the future.

It may be that neither you nor your partner expects the father to be deeply affected psychologically by the pregnancy, but he, too, is troubled by ambivalence and anxiety about the impending changes. He may resent the physical effects on you of nausea and fatigue. He may feel pride coupled with a heavy sense of responsibility to provide for his offspring and his mate, which can be less threatening to an older father who is financially secure. Like his partner, the man is forced to examine his relationship with his own parent, while coming to grips with his image of himself as a father. Beset by this unexpected turmoil, your partner finds himself called on to support you. Even more than a woman, a man is likely to deny or suppress feelings of self-doubt and fear, not recognizing them as normal and common. Many societies deal with this problem by practicing *couvade*, a way of involving the father in the pregnancy by prescribing certain conduct for him. The expectant father may have to adopt a special diet, avoid foods such as meat, fish, or salt, and may have to eat alone and not cook anything himself. He may be barred from all but the most necessary work, or be forbidden to touch tools. The man may even manifest his mate's physical symptoms up to and including labor and delivery. Although *couvade* is not practiced in our society, *couvade* syndrome is not uncommon, in which your partner could actually experience some physical symptoms of pregnancy.

It's extremely important for you and your partner to recognize and discuss all your feelings. Suppressing and burying them will not make them go away; talking about them will help you assist each other in dealing with them. If your partner doesn't know about your insecurities and anxieties, he can't respond to them. If you turn so far inward that you don't notice your partner's upheaval, you fail to give him necessary support. A man who feels rejected, shut out, in the early months of pregnancy begins a withdrawal from his partner that may last well past delivery. Avoid this by staying open to each other.

Like your moods, your desire for sex will go up and down during pregnancy, as will your mate's. Sometimes these fluctuations will place the two of you on opposite ends of the scale. If you're experiencing considerable nausea and/or fatigue during these early months, expect it to interfere with your sexuality. If you've had a previous miscarriage, you may be very nervous about intercourse during this trimester. On the other hand, if you've been having sex on schedule as a means of achieving conception, you may feel liberated by your success and able to enjoy sexual relations in a relaxed way that hasn't been possible for some time. Similarly, if you always worried about getting pregnant during intercourse, you may enjoy sex more now that "the worst" has happened.

Contrary to many people's notions, sexual desire and response can be at least as great during pregnancy as at other times. Prohibitions against sexual intercourse and orgasm during pregnancy have been discarded, on the whole, as antibiotics have neutralized the threat of infection and more has become known about the physiology involved. There are still instances when intercourse is inadvisable (when, for example, the woman has an incompetent cervix), but on the whole, your practitioner isn't likely to set any limits. This freedom does not necessarily extend to the immediate postpartum period, however, when your interest in sex is likely to be strictly minimal anyway. Do discuss any questions either of you have with your practitioner, and do confide in each other about your changing sexual needs. You will have to make adjustments throughout the pregnancy to remain mutually satisfied, and you can't make the right ones if you don't understand each other's needs.

Prenatal Care in Early Pregnancy

It is especially crucial for an older mother, who is some-what more likely to have a preexisting medical condition or to develop certain complications in her pregnancy, to initiate prompt prenatal care. It's only common sense that serious problems can best be treated when diagnosed early on. And minor problems can be kept minor or eliminated if they're not given a chance to develop. Make an appointment to confirm pregnancy when your period is a few weeks overdue, and begin prenatal care.

At your first prenatal visit, your entire medical history will be recorded. Following that, a fairly thorough physical examination is done. You'll be asked to urinate first, and the urine will be tested for a variety of abnormal substances including sugar, protein, and blood. You'll be weighed and asked if this is your prepregnant weight; your height will be measured, your blood pressure and pulse checked.

During the physical examination, the practitioner will evaluate your general appearance and state of health and will examine your skin, eyes, ears, nose, throat, thyroid, breasts, heart and lung sounds, abdomen, lymph nodes, arms, and legs. You'll be checked for swelling and have a neurological exam. Your practitioner will try to feel the uterus in the abdomen, although that's not usually possible until about 12 weeks. During the pelvic exam, your practitioner will usually tell you if your uterus is enlarged and how much so; that is, if your period is two weeks overdue, he or she may say the uterus is six-week size. Your cervix will be examined for color (bluish when pregnant, pink when not), consistency, bleeding, inflammation, and old scars and to be sure the opening, or os, is closed. Aspects of the vagina and external genitals will also be examined. Your pelvis will be measured, if it is small, the possibility of a cesarean delivery might be discussed now. A Pap smear is often done at the time of the pelvic exam. A rectal exam finishes the procedure.

Laboratory tests in conjunction with your first visit include urinalysis and possibly a test to confirm your pregnancy. Some blood work is also done, to make sure you are not anemic, to check for any possible blood incompatabilities between you and your child, and to establish the Rh type. If you're Rh negative and the baby is Rh positive, it's possible that antibodies in your blood will attack your baby's red blood cells containing the Rh substance. Your blood will be checked throughout your pregnancy to be sure it's not manufacturing Rh antibodies; if it is, an intrauterine transfusion may be needed. Injection of a substance called RhoGAM after delivery or miscarriage prevents formation of the antibodies in future pregnancies.

You will also routinely be checked for syphilis and for immunity to rubella (German measles). Other laboratory tests may be ordered for particular problems. Occasionally, if there is a question as to whether you are indeed pregnant or if you have been spotting, ultrasound will be ordered at this time. The ultrasound procedure is described in the following chapter on second trimester pregnancy.

After the physical exam is a good time to ask questions, such as what the costs will be. An obstetrician or midwife usually charges a flat fee for the whole package, from initial visit through postpartum checkup, with extra fees for special services, such as a cesarean delivery, and tests, such as ultrasound and amniocentesis. The practitioner can also tell you what the hospital charges are likely to be.

During this first prenatal visit, you should, if you haven't done so previously, establish a good rapport with the practitioner(s) who will be following you. The first visit is usually a long one, since it involves so much questioning, examining, and testing. (Your choice of practitioner and obstetric care is discussed in detail in Chapter 8.) Buy a small notebook and bring it with you to this visit; in it, jot down all the questions you and your partner have for your practitioner and the answers you're given. Continue to jot down questions as they occur to you and your partner throughout your pregnancy, and bring the notebook with you to each prenatal visit. Also record your symptoms in the notebook so you'll remember to report them at your next visit.

Because so much information is given about your pregnancy at the first visit, and because you may just now be getting acquainted with the person who will most likely deliver your child, it is a good idea for your partner to join you. He, too, will have many questions which may be best answered directly. He is also likely to feel somewhat left out of the pregnancy, especially during the first trimester, when few of the myriad changes going on in your body are visible to him. Joining you at the first prenatal visit allows him to participate and can make both of you feel less as though this is something happening to you alone.

You will probably be given your due date on this first visit, but you can also figure it out for yourself. Begin on day 1 of your last menstrual period, count ahead 9 months, and add 7 days; this is your expected date of delivery. It can, however, often vary 2 weeks in either direction and still be considered completely normal. In fact, pregnancy usually lasts 40 weeks, yet these days a baby is not considered premature after 36 weeks are completed.

After an evaluation of your present health and your apparent risk factors, the next prenatal visit will be set up. If you have no particular problems, it may be a month or even six weeks between visits in the early part of your pregnancy.

Often, by your second prenatal visit, the first trimester is almost over. Finishing a trimester—especially the first—is a real milestone. Your pregnancy is one third completed, yet most people looking at you still won't realize you're pregnant. If you've been feeling lousy during the first trimester, there's an excellent chance you'll perk up during the second. And a spontaneous abortion becomes much less likely once the first trimester is over.

CHAPTER 4

THE SECOND TRIMESTER OF PREGNANCY

The second trimester of your pregnancy—the fourth, fifth, and sixth months—is a period in which both you and the outside world become unmistakably aware of the developing baby inside you. It's a period of exciting changes—your early-pregnancy nausea and fatigue will almost certainly vanish, you'll switch to maternity clothes, the whole world will know you're pregnant, and your baby will show unmistakable signs of life.

Fetal Development in the Second Three Months

During these three months, the fetus grows from a one-ounce, 3-inch scrap of life to a two-pound, 14-inch nearly viable human being. The rapid formation in the first trimester of organs and systems has given way to growth. During the fourth month, the fetus develops a skeleton. Hair begins to grow all over the body and more organs start to function. Blood vessels just under the skin make the fetus bright pink. It is now six inches long and weighs four to six ounces.

By the end of the fifth fetal month, fine downy hair called lanugo covers the baby. Hair also grows on the head. The skin is very wrinkled, because no fat pads have yet developed. The fetus has begun to swallow some amniotic fluid, which is processed by the kidneys. The baby's arm and leg movements have become strong enough to be felt by you. From now on the baby will grow much more rapidly than its nourisher, the placenta.

The fetus has grown to 10 inches in length, weighs about a pound, and looks like a miniature baby or a subminiature old man.

After six months, a creamy white substance called vernix covers the baby's skin, to protect it from the amniotic fluid. Imagine what your skin would look like after being immersed in water for nine months without protection! The skin is a bit less wrinkled, because fat is being produced. The proportion of the head to the rest of the body is decreasing. The baby is now about 15 inches long and weighs two to two and a half pounds. There is some chance of survival outside the uterus now if the baby gets expert intensive care. That's a big change from the end of the first trimester!

Changes and Common Complaints of Middle Pregnancy

Dramatic changes are happening to you, too. Perhaps the most dramatic is the change in your body shape. As you looked in the mirror during the first trimester, you may have seen a riper, more voluptuous edition of yourself, but not an obviously pregnant person. As you continue to watch your mirror image in the course of these middle three months, you'll see your waistline disappear and your belly round out. The uterus expands and rises; by the time you are 20 weeks it will be approximately at your naval, and will be an inch or two higher after another month. It will also weigh 20 times what it used to. Your blood volume will have expanded by up to 50%. This, plus the growth of the fetus and placenta, accounts for a noticeable weight gain.

Your bathroom scale may have registered a small gain in the first trimester. Your weight will, of course, continue to increase, so it won't be long before your regular clothes can no longer accommodate the growing weight and the expanding bulge in your abdomen. During your fifth month (or sooner, if you've been pregnant before), you'll most likely switch to maternity clothes. The need to do so, however, comes for each of us at a slightly different time. In general, the body contours remain closer to the norm longer in the first pregnancy than in subsequent ones. Don't try to squeeze into your regular clothes for too long. They'll bind and be uncomfortable and, most important, you'll end up looking and feeling dumpy.

Finding suitable maternity clothes luckily isn't as hard as it used to be. You may still be confronted by an array of little-girlish, horribly cute garments that are totally inappropriate if you're over 35. I was particularly repelled by designers' insistence on short, puffed sleeves, frilly bows, and smocked tops that seemed to ape childhood dresses. Fortunately, most maternity stores now carry many clothes that look like what you'd normally wear—jeans, active sportswear, grown-up separates, and clothes suitable for the workplace. If you don't see what you want, try ordering by mail; department stores and maternity shops commonly issue catalogues for this purpose. Don't buy everything all at once; it will be refreshing as your pregnancy progresses to add some new clothes when you begin to get bored with your body image. Buying or at least dressing in new clothes is always fun!

Think in terms of recycling them after birth. At first you won't ever want to look at your maternity clothes again, but many blouses and dresses can be worn and look good postpregnancy by adding a belt or sash. I once turned a blouse into a beach jacket. For a winter pregnancy, try long nonmaternity cardigan sweaters; you may not be able to button them now, but they'll be great the following year. Some maternity clothes are now made to be recycled; you can buy skirts and jeans with adjustable closures to fit through pregnancy and for years afterward.

Some nonmaternity clothes can also be worn while you're pregnant. When the "big look" is in fashion, flowing dresses and tops may be spacious enough to fit for most of the nine months. Your partner's shirts and sweaters may be quite suitable for casual wear. Capes can take the place of fitted coats.

Stylish maternity clothes aren't cheap, especially for the working woman who requires such pricey items as suits and silk blouses. But you may not have to buy many. Maternity clothes seem to be passed around endlessly; friends and relatives will offer you their temporarily or permanently retired wardrobes, which will probably include some garments from *their* friends and relatives. One of my friends gave birth, unexpectedly, wearing my favorite maternity sundress! Another friend remarked that she'd never been so well dressed, at home and at the office, as when she was pregnant, thanks to the multitude of clothes lent to her. Secondhand maternity shops are another source of inexpensive apparel.

You'll probably have to buy new underwear. Your growing breasts will push you into a larger bra size or prompt you to wear a bra when you haven't before. If you wear bikini panties normally, you may find as I did that they'll fit all through your pregnancy, gradually disappearing from view below your expanding uterus; otherwise you'll have to buy maternity panties that fit over your abdomen. In either case, they should have a cotton crotch, since you are more susceptible to vaginal infections while pregnant and need the nonitching, ventilating properties of cotton rather than nylon.

Once you're into maternity clothes, be prepared for people to react differently toward you. Total strangers will notice you, ask when you're due, comment on your size, tell you about their niece's pregnancy, even pat your belly. Obviously, some people feel that pregnancy belongs in part to society as a whole, not just to the mother, and so behavior that would be considered grossly rude for the nonpregnant woman is more or less acceptable for the pregnant one. I never got quite used to this. You may expect family and perhaps close friends to take a proprietary view of your pregnancy, but not strangers or remote acquaintances. You and your partner may welcome this attention or find it downright unpleasant; still, you might as well accept it, because it will follow you until delivery.

It's not just your expanding midsection and new wardrobe that make your pregnancy a reality for you and your partner during the second trimester. You also get concrete evidence of the presence of a live being inside you. Sometime early in the second trimester you can listen to your baby's heartbeat with the Doppler, a kind of electronic stethoscope placed on your abdomen. It's very exciting when you first hear it—there really is something alive in there!—and it remains exciting as well as reassuring on each prenatal visit. The baby's heart beats much faster than yours and has a different character, with a rapid whoo-whoo sound. Using a regular stethoscope, the baby's heartbeat may not be heard until the 20th week, or about halfway through your pregnancy.

The other evidence of your baby's life, and probably the most thrilling event of the second trimester, comes when you begin to feel the baby move inside you. This also happens around the 20th week, although in a second pregnancy you'll recognize the early sensations of fetal movement about two weeks earlier. You'll feel some vague flutterings or twitches in your stomach and wonder for a week or two if it's gas rumbling around. As the sensations continue and get stronger, you will realize that it's your baby kicking and flailing about. By the sixth month, you and your partner can see your abdomen move, and you can both feel the baby's prods and kicks when you place a hand on your stomach.

The second trimester is often referred to as the "quiet" period of pregnancy, which it may be for your obstetrician, but isn't really for you. The nausea of the first trimester has most likely passed, and you may find yourself possessed of an amazing appetite. I shocked myself and my mother-in-law, who had been urging food on me for years, the night I lifted my five-month-pregnant body from the dinner table and announced I was going out to the kitchen for a first-ever second helping. While you were sleepy and tired during the first three months, all of a sudden, you'll be energetic now. The lifting of the uterus has taken pressure off your bladder, so you'll urinate less frequently. Both you and your partner will probably have come to terms with the fact of your pregnancy so you'll be calmer and more relaxed. You're not yet large enough to feel uncomfortable or awkward, so there's little restriction of your normal activities. This is the time to accomplish projects you'll find difficult later in pregnancy or when you have an infant to care for.

As you become demonstrably pregnant, you may wonder if travel must be restricted. It's perfectly okay during a normal pregnancy, but you do need to break up long trips every few hours to walk around, stretch, and keep the circulation flowing in your legs. Pillows or other soft padding tucked behind your back or under your legs will help alleviate cramps and aches. Travel very late in pregnancy may be inadvisable—you don't want to deliver your baby in unfamiliar, untested surroundings, especially if you've planned your birth setting very carefully. Some airlines require a letter from your obstetrician stating your due date and giving you medical clearance to fly, and some do not permit a woman very near term to fly at all. Check with your carrier before arriving at the gate with an eight- or nine-month-size belly. Do not fly in a nonpressurized aircraft.

Although you'll feel generally healthy during the second

trimester, there are some causes for grumbling. You may experience some of them or none of them, or they may crop up earlier or later in your pregnancy.

Pregnancy "Glow"

You may have heard of the "glow" of pregnancy. This is not just a myth. It can make you look better but at the same time make you feel uncomfortable. Your blood volume has expanded by 40% and your metabolism has also increased. Your skin is dissipating extra heat, and it's flushed and warm from the expanded blood vessels in it. You feel warm to the touch, you get easily overheated, and you're perspiring more. Your nails and hair grow faster. There's not much you can do about this other than wear lightweight, somewhat loose-fitting clothes and avoid overheated, stuffy interiors.

Breathlessness

As the uterus expands upward toward the diaphragm and the abdomen extends outward, the lungs are cramped and can't expand as fully. At the same time, your body needs more oxygen. Thus, breathlessness is a common and normal symptom that often appears in the second trimester. If you do heavy exercise or physical labor, you may feel the need to slow down because your breathing can't keep pace with your exertions. If you are a runner, you may find yourself feeling better at a fast walk. Your body is giving you the correct message. Good posture, pulling in on the abdomen, will allow the lungs a bit more space.

Backache

Backache, too, is a normal discomfort of pregnancy which sometimes tends to become more bothersome as you move closer to term. The joints in your pelvis and spine soften and loosen during pregnancy, and you also have a new center of gravity. This makes you more susceptible to back injury, which is why you're supposed to avoid lifting or moving heavy objects just now. Several things can bring relief. Sleep on a firm mattress, supplemented if necessary by a sheet of plywood. Concentrate on good posture all the time; keeping your spine straight can help a lot. Wear low-heeled shoes. Exercise daily in moderation, to strengthen the back muscles. See your practitioner or prepared-childbirth instructor for specific routines, such as the basic pelvic rock, in which you tilt your pelvis forward, flatten your back, and tighten your abdomen and buttocks. You can do this lying down, sitting, standing, or on hands and knees. I found daily pelvic rock exercises, as well as a heating pad and light back massage, very effective.

Headache

Headache plagues some women during pregnancy. It is particularly annoying if you are simultaneously experiencing nausea or general malaise. Unfortunately, you have only two choices: suffer or take it lying down. Check with your doctor before taking any medication; aspirin, for instance, may seem perfectly safe to you, but it can be just the opposite. Severe persistent headache, especially in the last trimester, should be reported.

Heartburn

Heartburn, which often occurs in the second trimester, can get progressively worse as the months go on. It results from gastric contents backing up into the esophagus due to a pro-gesterone-relaxed muscle at the top of the stomach and is probably aggravated by pressure from the growing uterus displacing abdominal contents. While heartburn doesn't count as a serious medical problem, it certainly can be unpleasant. Lying down or bending over makes it worse. Sipping tea, chewing gum, wearing looser clothes and switching to a more upright sleeping position using several pillows might soothe you. Again, be sure to check with your doctor before trying any antacid; even plain old baking soda can be harmful because of its high sodium content.

Varicose Veins and Hemorrhoids

Varicose veins in the legs and hemorrhoids, enlarged veins in the rectal opening, can both cause considerable discomfort and tend to become more problematic with subsequent pregnancies. They are both related to increased circulation and increased pressure from the enlarging uterus. In the case of hemorrhoids, the pregnancy-expanded rectal veins are further strained by constipation. The best treatment for hemorrhoids is prevention—see the suggestions for constipation in the section on complaints of first trimester pregnancy. If necessary, a safe stool softener can be prescribed for you. A warm-tub soak or a cold witch-hazel compress can relieve discomfort and promote shrinkage. The more weight you put on, the more severe the problem is likely to become; you cannot help gaining, but you should make an effort to observe the guidelines recommended for your pregnancy.

Varicose veins are initiated or promoted by the increased quantity of blood pooling in your legs. Heredity can predispose you to varicose veins, both before and during pregnancy, and if you have them while carrying one child, you're likely to have them again in your next pregnancy. The problem will get better postpartum, but it may not disappear entirely. To avoid or alleviate varicose veins, try to improve circulation in your legs. Don't sit or stand in one spot for long periods of time. Have nothing constricting around your legs, like tight pants or elastic-top hose, and be sure to walk around a fair amount every day. Elevate your legs at intervals. Keep your feet raised on a stool or low chair when you're sitting, and don't cross your legs. As with hemorrhoids, control weight gain. You can be fitted for special stretch stockings if necessary. Hot, reddened areas or streaks, lines, or a knot on either leg should be reported immediately.

Swelling

Some swelling, especially of the ankles and feet, is routine in pregnancy. Your tissues, stimulated by the pregnancy hormones, retain extra fluid, a condition you may also have noticed in the days just before your period started, or if you were ever on the Pill. Gravity causes some of this fluid to settle in your lower legs. Hands and fingers may also swell. The last months of pregnancy and hot weather aggravate the condition. To alleviate it, you should wear open shoes and do leg- and arm-raising exercises several times daily. If you notice your fingers swelling, take off your rings while you still can. If your salt intake is heavy, cut back, but don't eliminate it entirely. Do mention the swelling to your practitioner, so he or she can check to be sure it's within normal limits.

Gas Pains

Gas, stomach cramps, and a distended abdomen may also crop up during the second trimester. These problems are usually made worse by big meals, carbonated beverages, and fats.

Also avoid anything that causes you gas normally and eat slowly. Exercise and avoiding long periods in any one position should help.

Cavities grow faster during pregnancy, and gums tend to swell and even to bleed, so pay special attention to brushing teeth and flossing. It's a good idea to have a dental checkup early in the second trimester, but don't have dental X-rays (see Chapter 7).

Don't be shy about reporting your discomforts; all deserve to be properly evaluated, and the people who are caring for you may have additional suggestions and recommend further testing or monitoring. You're helping your practitioner by reporting all your symptoms, and you're also quelling any anxiety you or your partner may feel because of them. Sometimes well-meaning but not necessarily knowledgeable friends and relatives either falsely reassure you or scare you unnecessarily. Also, if this is your second or higher pregnancy, you may feel you shouldn't have questions because you've been through it all before. But more often than not, each pregnancy, like each child, is different, bringing with it different symptoms and concerns you'll want to ask about.

Psychological and Sexual Changes of Middle Pregnancy

Psychologically, things should smooth out during the second trimester. You emerge from your self-absorbed state and begin dealing with the outside world's reactions to you as a pregnant person. If it's not your first pregnancy, you may be disappointed in the decreased interest shown by others as compared with the first time around. My friend Kate complained that her parents took the announcement of her second child's conception so casually, she wasn't even sure they'd understood what she had told them! You may be reluctant to commit yourself emotionally to the pregnancy until after you've been given the results of your amniocentesis, around the 20th week.

Nevertheless, in all likelihood you are no longer ambivalent as in the early months; your partner, however, may well be. Researcher Katharyn A. May has identified three phases of father involvement in pregnancy: the announcement phase, when pregnancy is first suspected and confirmed; the moratorium phase, when men cease consciously thinking about the pregnancy; and the focusing phase, when the father feels the reality of the pregnancy (*Nursing Research*, November/December 1982). Your partner may be in his moratorium for much of the second trimester, just when you are turning to him, seeking his support, enthusiasm, participation. Don't push him for involvement yet if he isn't ready. According to May, the emotional distancing, which can last for several months, seems to allow a man time to accept the pregnancy as a reality and as a positive event. The more ready a man is for pregnancy, the shorter the moratorium period, so older fathers may have an advantage: increased financial security and a stable partnership boost pregnancy readiness. This on-hold emotional period usually ends when the pregnancy becomes obvious.

Because attention focuses on you, it's important to remember that your partner may feel jealous and left out. Pay close attention to his needs now; continue a reasonable number of joint social and recreational activities; when he's ready, start to prepare for the baby, together. This should come naturally for you, because your partner is a ready focus of your new outer-directedness. A man who is feeling shut out or who is seeking to avoid the pregnancy will plunge into other activities—business trips, late nights at the office, sports, even other women. He won't necessarily recognize why he is doing this. The pattern of behavior should be noticed and discussed so the reasons for it can be dealt with.

As you negotiate the level of your partner's involvement during this trimester, you'll be led toward an ongoing discussion of parenting roles, particularly the degree of father involvement. What's important is to achieve similar expectations. *JOGN Nursing* (September/October 1984) reports that expectant fathers' anxiety levels correlate with agreement between parents on the father's role, mutual expectations equalling lowered anxiety; a high projected childcare level for the father does not increase anxiety if both parents agree on the role. Again, age and higher income are advantages, predisposing couples to greater agreement on the father's role.

While your body enlarges, both you and your partner must

adjust to your new temporary physical shape. It is unsettling, for both of you. Nevertheless, you may feel more erotic now, especially since the physical discomforts of early pregnancy have eased. Your partner, however, may be less interested in sex than when you were in your first trimester. Some men are turned off by their partner's body changes, while others find them sexually stimulating. If the baby is active during your sexual activity, either or both of you may find that disturbing. Fears of harming the baby during intercourse may surface. It is quite rare that sexual relations during pregnancy are anything but perfectly safe, but if you need reassurance, discuss your fears with your practitioner.

Prenatal Care in Middle Pregnancy

Providing no special problems develop, you'll probably see your practitioner once a month during the second trimester. These visits are quite short, consisting of routine checkups.

AFP Testing

Several special tests may be done during the second trimester. Around your 16th week, or anytime between the 12th and 20th weeks, a blood sample may be taken to check your alpha fetoprotein levels. AFP is produced by the fetus and passes into your bloodstream. Exceptionally high levels— found in only 1% of women tested—can indicate normal multiple pregnancy as well as neural tube defects (for example, spina bifida or anencephaly), which are rare but very serious fetal abnormalities of the developing spinal cord, brain, and backbone. Ultrasound and amniocentesis (discussed in the following sections) can confirm the presence of abnormalities suggested by AFP results. AFP may also be tested as part of amniocentesis.

Ultrasound

Ultrasound, also called sonography, is a diagnostic tool that may be used anytime during pregnancy to confirm or rule out suspected problems. It's always performed prior to amniocentesis. It bounces sound waves (not radiation) off your internal structures; the resulting impulses are displayed on a kind of snowy TV screen. Sonography can be used to diagnose pregnancy, to monitor fetal and placental growth, to reveal fetal malformations, to confirm the presence of multiple fetuses, and to verify fetal age. Later in pregnancy, ultrasound can be used to determine if the baby's head is too large for the mother's pelvis, to show whether a placental abnormality has developed, or to establish the baby's position.

The procedure itself only takes about 20 to 30 minutes. First you must drink a lot of fluids to fill the bladder. This is usually the only uncomfortable part—you just don't have much room for a full bladder when you're pregnant. An ultrasound scan may be done at your doctor's office or at a medical center. The image on the screen will look somewhat fuzzy to you, but the technician and/or physician performing the scan will point out the different structures to you. If he or she doesn't explain the picture, ask! The picture can be difficult for untrained persons to interpret. Marcia was horrified to hear a young nurse exclaim at the ultrasound image, "Doctor, there's one body and two heads!" The nurse had misidentified uterine fibroids; the fetus was in fact completely normal, as Marcia's physician hastily assured her.

Doctors consider ultrasound to be, on the whole, safe and noninvasive—a wonderful diagnostic tool. There is no evidence that it's ever been harmful to humans. Nevertheless, there is some controversy about its use. *Lancet*, an authoritative British medical journal, reported in November 1984 the conclusions of two surveys of children who had been exposed to ultrasound in utero. Newspaper headlines read, "Ultrasound Found Safe in Pregnancy," but the findings referred only to cancer. No link was found between the exposure and childhood cancer, including leukemia. However, cellular changes have been found in laboratory animals after ultrasound exposure, and there is still no conclusive proof that ultrasound has no deleterious delayed effects, as X-rays were found to have. For this reason, ultrasound isn't used routinely, for all pregnancies. The National Institutes of Health recommend that sonography be used during pregnancy only for specific medical reasons, of which it lists 28.

Amniocentesis

Because you're over 35, your prenatal routine will differ from younger women's in one important respect: amniocentesis will be discussed. Your practitioner will probably recommend it, and you may well opt for it. As I will explain in Chapter 6, one serious risk dramatically increases with maternal age: the risk of conceiving a fetus with a chromosomal abnormality. The most common is Down's syndrome (mongolism). Since Down's and many other chromosomal abnormalities can be diagnosed by testing the amniotic fluid, this testing is likely to be recommended to you. And due to the plethora of malpractice suits, your practitioner is certain to discuss the procedure with you.

A new procedure of testing for fetal defects called chorionic villus sampling which is not yet routinely used is also discussed in Chapter 6.

Because amniocentesis carries some risk of spontaneous abortion (see below), medical personnel vary in the degree to which they recommend the procedure; some advocate that every woman aged 35 or more should have the test, while others don't believe chromosomal risks make the test necessary until a woman is 37 or 38. Genetic counselors favor the procedure at least by the age of 35. Pregnant women vary a lot, too, in their decisions to go ahead with the testing or skip it. The women I interviewed were certainly not agreed. For example, several opted against amniocentesis because they felt they wouldn't terminate the pregnancy in any event. Barbara declined the testing at age 38 but felt she would have done it at 40. Karen, 35, wouldn't take the chance of disturbing the pregnancy because she'd had many previous miscarriages. So had Marcia, 39, but she did take the risk, although unlike Karen, she already had two children. Laura, 35, chose to be tested although her doctor advised against it at her age; the doctor's wife did the same! I myself chose amniocentesis for both my pregnancies, at 36 and 40; I felt I did not have the emotional resources to care for a severely handicapped child.

Both a genetic counselor and the director of maternal–fetal medicine at a major medical center with whom I spoke had the same comment: women who think they would not want an abortion under any circumstances change their minds in the vast majority of cases when they learn they are carrying a seriously deformed or abnormal child. This may be related to a phenomenon mentioned by genetic counselor Edward Kloza of Maine's Foundation for Blood Research: many women, although they know the statistics, don't really believe it could happen to them, that there is an actual risk to *this* child. So an initial unwillingness to abort may not be a reason to skip amniocentesis. Also, knowing that they are going to have a child with, say, Down's syndrome, gives a couple the opportunity to prepare themselves informationally and emotionally for that reality.

Statistically, according to the *American Journal of Obstetrics and Gynecology* (March 15, 1981), amniocentesis is used more by people with high educational levels, by white women, by higher-income couples, and by urban residents. It's used most routinely by women who work in the health or mental health profession (nurses, therapists, counselors who deal with retarded people and their families). These women have amniocentesis in the early or mid 30's—even in their 20's—to alleviate the anxiety caused by their knowledge of just how devastating it is to deal with severe retardation on a daily basis.

Overall, 50% to 60% of women over 35 elect amniocentesis when offered it. You may find that amniocentesis is not routinely done in your area for women who are 35 or 36, but the reason is sometimes practical rather than medical. Where laboratory facilities are overburdened, the age limits for routine amniocentesis are sometimes raised. You should still be able to have the testing done, but you may have to insist.

Amniocentesis is done either at your doctor's office or in a medical center to which your doctor sends you. It is often preceded by genetic counseling, especially if done at a medical center. You'll also be referred for genetic counseling if you've previously had a child born with an abnormality. The counselor will explain to you and your partner what problems can be revealed by prenatal diagnosis and what disorders you may be at risk for because of your age or other factors. Total costs including doctor, counselor, radiologist, hospital, and lab fees average $800.

Usually, amniocentesis is done at 16 weeks (before then there is insufficient fluid), but it takes 3 or 4 weeks to get the results. The procedure is fairly simple. First, ultrasound delineates the position of the baby, the placenta, and other structures; measurements taken from this will quite accurately determine fetal age. Next, you'll probably be given local anesthesia. Then a needle is inserted through your abdomen and through the uterine wall into the amniotic fluid surrounding the baby. Less than an ounce of fluid is drawn out. The ultrasound picture shows the doctor where to put the needle to avoid jabbing any important structures.

The procedure doesn't take too long. It hurts a bit as the uterus contracts in response to the needle and it is a little scary. I wanted my husband with me both times, and the medical personnel didn't mind. Most women do bring their husbands; a calm, nonqueasy, supportive person helps. Gail (37) brought her 11-year-old son, too, so he could see the ultrasound picture of his sibling-to-be.

The aspirated fluid is sent to a laboratory, where the fetal cells found in the fluid are allowed to grow. Only after they have multiplied can they be analyzed, which is why it takes four weeks for you to get the results. The cells' chromosomes are studied, and blood and enzyme abnormalities can also be detected. Testing of the amniotic fluid after the cells have been removed is a separate procedure, not always done. These fluid studies include AFP testing, which can reveal a serious abnormality such as spina bifida. Discuss this with your practitioner. If you aren't having blood AFP screening, you will probably want to be sure your amniocentesis includes both a cell culture and a fluid study.

Perhaps the hardest part of amniocentesis is waiting for the results. You want to know that everything's okay, yet you dread finding out it's not. Most women expect to test out normally, and in the overwhelming majority of cases, they do. The odds are very much on your side that everything is fine. A chart in Chapter 6 shows this. Of course, if an abnormality is found, you'll have to discuss it thoroughly with your doctor or genetic counselor. She or he can provide you with all the available information on the condition so you can make a decision to terminate or not based on sound, expert advice. Unfortunately, you'll be 20 weeks pregnant by now—halfway along, and showing. A decision to terminate can prove very difficult at this stage and carries with it the necessity of explaining what's happened to all of those people who've known you're pregnant.

While techniques have become quite refined, amniocentesis can occasionally induce a spontaneous abortion. A figure often quoted is 1 abortion out of every 200 cases, but the risks today are probably lower than that. Elsa Reich, a genetic coun-

selor at New York University School of Medicine, advises her
patients that their risk of miscarriage following amniocentesis is
1 out of 300; other counselors and medical centers quote figures
from 1 out of 200 to 1 out of 350. Some practitioners feel these
risks are too high compared with the chances of conceiving a
child with Down's syndrome at the age of 35 or 36, so they
don't routinely recommend amniocentesis until 37 or older. Yet
despite this recommendation, that only women past 37 have
routine amniocentesis testing in order to minimize the risk to a
probably-healthy fetus, many women 34, 35 or 36 are still more
willing to take a chance of harming that fetus than of carrying a
severely retarded child. These women will opt for the test
despite its risks rather than suffer the dire consequences of
giving birth to a Down's child.

Another serious but rare complication of amniocentesis is
the possibility of infection and injury to the fetus or placenta.
Less serious problems involve difficulties in obtaining the fluid
and culturing the cells, especially in the case of fraternal twins
with two amniotic sacs to locate and draw from. It's best to have
the procedure performed by an experienced practitioner and
the analysis itself done at a center that handles a large number
of these tests. Minor symptoms that you might experience after
the test are mild cramping, discomfort, and slight leakage of
fluid. Any severe pains, fever, or vaginal leakage should of
course be reported.

Amniocentesis does carry one interesting side result: the
chromosome study reveals the sex of your baby. Sometimes
you can even see the baby's sex on the sonogram. You'll be
asked if you want to be told; knowing that it's knowable makes
it awfully hard to say no. You can gear yourself up emotionally
for whatever sex child you're going to have and avoid disap-
pointment when the baby's born. You can prepare your friends
and relatives, if you want to, or you can enjoy keeping them
guessing. And you only have to think of one name. Soon you
may be able to know the sex of your baby without undergoing
amniocentesis: the August '84 issue of *Vogue* magazine reported that a gender test kit will soon be on sale in drugstores,
for accurate gender identification after you're six months pregnant.

CHAPTER 5

THE THIRD TRIMESTER OF PREGNANCY

The final three months of pregnancy can seem interminable. A friend of mine begged her doctor to induce labor the moment she reached term, unable to bear the thought of being overdue. Her age, 36, may have played a role in her impatience. She really wanted to get on with things. You too may await the first labor pain like a sign from heaven.

Fetal Development in the Last Three Months

This is the period during which your baby develops fat deposits under the skin, loses the wrinkles, and acquires a new-baby-like appearance, adding a lot of weight to your already burgeoning body. After seven months, the fetus weighs up to four pounds and measures close to 16 inches. It is storing iron, fat, and more calcium. If it's a boy, his testes begin to descend. The lungs begin to mature. Should the baby be born at the end of seven months, he or she will be weak but have a good chance of survival with expert supportive care.

By the end of eight months, the baby weighs five pounds or more and measures up to 18 inches. More iron and calcium have been stored, as well as nitrogen, and a lot of fat has been deposited under the thickening skin. The organs and nervous system are nearly mature and are functioning. Usually the baby gets into the final, head-down position before the ninth month starts.

During the ninth month, your baby continues to add fat, gain weight, and become rounder. The head settles down further into your pelvis. The red skin turns pink. Most of the lanugo, the downy hair that covers the fetus, is shed; if it is still present at birth, it will soon disappear. The creamy vernix that covers the fetal skin is decreasing; what's left after birth will be wiped off. When you see your baby, she or he will most likely have some scalp hair, plus well-developed fingernails and toe-nails—they may even need trimming! At birth, most babies weigh between six and nine pounds and are 19 to 20 inches long. Babies born from 36 to 41 weeks are considered term; before then they are preterm, and after that they are postterm.

Changes and Common Complaints of Late Pregnancy

During the third trimester, you begin to think of your body as not your own. You wonder who it is you see in the mirror with that incredible shape. You make jokes, which aren't *all* that funny to you, about losing sight of your toes. You are physically forced to slow down because your body is getting bigger and clumsier. Some women even outgrow their less voluminous maternity clothes and need their partner's help to roll over in bed!

During the first and for a good part of the second trimester, you will probably not have gained much weight. This will change in the last part of the second trimester and during the third one, when you'll add about a pound a week.

In your last three months, your breathing will grow more rapid and you might find yourself short of breath. Your heart rate will also increase somewhat. As you get nearer to term, your blood pressure will rise. The height of your uterus will increase about half an inch per week. You'll be very conscious of your baby's moving around, which can be both a pleasure and a discomfort. You may be able to identify your baby's head and bottom by feeling your abdomen; your practitioner at your prenatal visits can help you do this.

Sometime early in the seventh month or late in the sixth, you and your partner will probably start prepared childbirth classes. You want to start early enough to accommodate a pre-due-date delivery, but not so early that you'll lose interest in practicing the techniques you've learned while you're waiting for labor to begin. For more information on prepared childbirth, see Chapter 8.

As with the earlier months of pregnancy, certain minor discomforts are associated with the third trimester, although they may crop up sooner. Or you may experience some of the complaints described in the second trimester now. Being over 35, you have a greater likelihood of developing varicose veins and hemorrhoids in the last trimester. Valves in the veins function less well with age; when significant uterine pressure further impedes circulation, varicose veins are likely to form in the legs. Working at a sedentary desk job for many years combines with pregnancy-related conditions to make you more prone to hemorrhoids.

Pressure and Pains

Feelings of sagging, heaviness, or dragging are fairly standard in the final months of pregnancy. Pressure on the pelvic structures and the abdomen naturally increases as the uterus expands. Lying on your side for short periods may help to relieve pressure, especially with pillows strategically placed—under your knees or chest, for instance, or tucked up against the small of your back. Sit cross-legged, tailor fashion, whenever possible; this tilts the uterus away from the back and eases pressure on the pelvis and the blood vessels to the legs. Practice exercises recommended by your practitioner or childbirth instructor to strengthen muscles, especially the abdominal ones. If necessary, wear a maternity girdle.

You may also experience some rib or chest pain caused by fetal pressure on the rib cage and muscle tension. Change position when you feel the pains, or raise your arms above your head and stretch.

Intermittent, irregular, relatively painless tightening of the uterus is quite common during the third trimester. You may have noticed these sensations, called Braxton-Hicks contractions, late in the second trimester. They increase in strength and frequency as you approach your due date. They are not true labor contractions and do not signal the onset of labor. They can be very annoying, especially if they interfere with your sleep, but they can't be prevented. Usually they go away when you get up and walk around. Strong, regular contractions that don't go away could be a sign of labor, premature or term, and should be reported.

Urinary Frequency

Frequent urination, which you experienced in the first trimester, sometimes returns to plague you during the final three months. As the baby and the uterus continue to expand, more and more pressure is placed on the bladder. You'll have to get up at night to urinate. You're likely to leak urine during vigorous exercise or hearty laughing. During my first pregnancy, I had to make a series of trips to a nearby courthouse to be authorized as a notary. Although it was only a half-hour drive from my house, I had to plan it around my insistent bladder. I simply could not make it without stopping at the Howard Johnson's along the way. I've never stopped there since!

Although you may be tempted to limit the amount of fluid you drink to cut down on the frequency of urination, it's not a good idea to do so. You need to keep your fluid intake levels relatively high. You can, however, limit caffeine; avoiding spices and alcohol may help. To help you sleep through the night, stay away from fluids after dinner, especially tea and coffee. If you develop burning or pain with urination, or cloudy or smelly urine, you may have an infection. Report the symptoms.

Leg Cramps

Another sleep interrupter that may develop is leg cramps. Nothing can jolt you out of a deep sleep better than a severe spasm in your calf. It's caused by sluggish circulation and a calcium imbalance. When you get a cramp, press your feet against a hard surface—the foot of the bed, the wall, the floor. To avoid cramps, practice leg-flexing exercises and increase your calcium intake. Vitamin B may help. Sleep with pillows under your legs and loose covers over them.

Leaking Nipples

In the weeks before your baby's birth, your breasts can produce so much colostrum—an opaque premilk fluid—that small amounts leak out the nipples. This is perfectly normal. Just rinse off your breasts periodically so the colostrum doesn't cake. You may need to use shields in your bra to protect your clothes from staining.

Stretch Marks

Stretch marks may also appear now. Not all women get them. They are caused by the separation of over-stretched tissue and the thinning out of the covering skin. Stretch marks occur where there is the most expansion: in the breasts and lower abdomen, and sometimes in the thighs. When they develop, they may be red or blue; over time, they fade to a silvery whitish tone. Hormones and heredity may influence your chances of developing these little scars. Rubbing the skin with rich lotions, natural oils, cocoa butter or, especially, vitamin E may help prevent or lessen stretch marks; even if it doesn't help, it can't hurt. Good posture, too, can reduce the stretching.

Fatigue

Another early pregnancy problem returns to bother you in the third trimester: fatigue. This time it's not caused by hormones but partially by simple lack of sleep. If Braxton-Hicks contractions don't wake you up, a leg cramp, a pressing need to urinate, or a strong poke in the ribs does. Your baby is so active, you wonder if he or she ever sleeps; the little devil seems to take your lying down as a signal to leap into action. The only solution is to nap during the day whenever you have a chance. At least you'll be used to interrupted sleep after the baby's born!

Fortunately, a lot of minor discomforts will ease during the ninth month. When the baby settles down into your pelvis, or becomes "engaged," you'll notice that your uterus appears much lower, or "dropped." Pressure on the lungs is relieved, easing your sense of breathlessness. You feel less enormous and awkward. There's a little more room in your stomach, and any rib and chest pains dissipate. Blood volume decreases slightly, so your heart isn't working quite as hard as it was. Since the baby is now more confined, you'll probably notice less fetal movement, which can be a relief after all the activity of the past few months. Once the baby has become engaged, if this is your first pregnancy, you can expect delivery in two to three weeks. In subsequent pregnancies, the baby may not engage until labor starts.

Psychological and Sexual Changes of Late Pregnancy

The psychological focus during the third trimester is on the imminent birth of your child. The physical process of labor and delivery lurks in your mind. Don't be surprised if you are fairly moody during the last trimester, elated as you mark off the weeks getting near term and alternately depressed and frustrated with an unwieldy body that is probably increasingly uncomfortable. Your whole body may seem more sensitive and reactive. You'll notice how thin everybody else looks and you may grow bored with your maternity clothes. A friend postulated that the last month of pregnancy and its attendant discomforts are nature's way of making us welcome labor! As a distraction, keep yourself active and busy, especially if you're overdue.

Since you are more physically stressed now than you were in the second trimester, you can expect accompanying mental pressure. This is a good time to start practicing stress-reduction techniques. Set aside some time, preferably more than once a day, for meditation, yoga, or relaxation techniques, quiet deep breathing and tension reduction. Exercises and sports are great stress relievers too.

Your partner will move into the focusing phase defined by May, mentioned in the previous chapter, during this trimester. The pregnancy will finally seem real to him; he'll focus on how he is experiencing it, and he will redefine himself as a father. As he becomes very interested in parents, children, and the daily impact of the pregnancy, he'll seem more supportive and considerate to you. He's likely to become very involved in practical preparations for the baby, like preparing the nursery. One terrific idea to foster this focusing is a baby shower for the father-to-be, with only men attending, including the expectant grandfathers.

Your partner can now shed his outsider's cloak and become an active participant. Childbirth classes call for a labor coach, who, in most cases, is the father. The coach plays a key role in prelabor practice, cueing relaxation and helping with exercises; the coach guides his partner through labor, acting as her support person, easing her discomfort, and helping her maintain her breathing and relaxation techniques. This active role can be especially appreciated by the expectant father who sees virtually the entire outside world centering its attention on his partner, while taking him for granted. Because the father's coaching role is so important, be sure he gets lots of sleep in the weeks before the baby is due, too. Neither of you wants to start labor exhausted.

Mutual preparation for childbirth can foster togetherness and mutual support. However, it's important for both of you to express honestly your feelings about father participation in labor and delivery. Some women genuinely don't want their husband present for delivery and are afraid to say so. Others say they don't, but only because they think that's their mate's unspoken preference. Some men want to help with labor but don't want to attend the delivery; they may feel unduly pressured to behave otherwise. Researcher Katharyn A. May found that many expectant fathers have what she calls an "observer style" (*Maternal Child Nursing*, September/October 1982). They do little prenatal decision making and remain somewhat detached throughout the pregnancy, although all but a few in May's study were supportive of their wives. These men reported being pressured and made to feel guilty by health professionals when they expressed reluctance to attend their wives' deliveries, although their partners accepted their hesitancy. Philip Taubman, writing in the *New York Times Magazine* (October 21, 1984), expressed his birth attendance experience this way: "I was truly astonished and awed. Yet, I wasn't sure I wanted to see my wife that way."

Talk openly about these emotions and the reasons for them to be sure you're not committing yourselves to a course that is psychologically inappropriate for either of you. Try attending at least one or two prepared childbirth classes together. Many men think they're reluctant to participate in labor and delivery but change their minds once they learn about what will happen. You may have to push to give your partner the opportunity. Tell him it is a proven fact that fathers who do participate tend to be more involved in childcare after the birth. Remember, too, that initial reluctance may dissipate once your partner reaches his focusing stage.

Couples have sexual intercourse less frequently toward the end of pregnancy, although this varies tremendously. Depending on the advice of your obstetrician or midwife, you can often have intercourse up until the time your membranes rupture, if there are no contraindications. This is not to say you'll necessarily feel like it or be comfortable during it. As your belly gets ever larger, you'll have to experiment to find new positions that aren't awkward. You might try a side-lying position with your partner behind you, rather like spoons. Any of a variety of noncoital methods can be mutually satisfying, too. You may find yourself and your partner much more in the mood for physical affection and not so interested in intercourse per se. Keep your minds and your communications open so you don't lose physical contact now.

Fears of infection and hurting the baby may resurface at this time, plus a worry that intercourse could trigger labor. It's true that maternal orgasm plus a hormone in sperm can cause uterine contractions, but this in turn doesn't precipitate labor in a normal pregnancy—unless you're at term, when it might, and then it's okay. The obstetrician of 37-year-old Valerie "prescribed" intercourse when she was three weeks overdue, to encourage labor to begin. If you have a history of prematurity, however, your practitioner may advise against intercourse during this trimester.

Prenatal Care in Late Pregnancy

Sometime during your seventh month, with no complications in sight, you'll begin having a prenatal visit every two weeks. This will switch to weekly during the ninth month. If you get much past your due date, you may be checked as often as every other day. An especially close watch will be kept on your blood pressure and urine if you're over 35, because the older woman has a propensity for high blood pressure and gestational diabetes (diabetes during pregnancy).

As prenatal visits get closer together in the later parts of pregnancy, the health professionals caring for you will usually give you progress reports about the position and approximate size of your baby, who is gaining almost a pound a week in the last month. Should there be a question about the baby's position or its size relative to your pelvis, you may have another ultrasound picture taken now.

Occasionally X-rays are used to measure the pelvis. Some

practitioners consider the procedure not too risky at this point in the pregnancy, because the dosage is so small and the fetus so well developed. Others, however, point to studies linking prenatal X-ray exposure and childhood leukemia and find little correlation between X-ray measure of pelvic size and eventual route of delivery (vaginal or cesarean). These practitioners discourage the use of X-ray pelvimetry.

A few weeks before delivery, you may be told about effacement and dilation. As the cervix gets ready for birth, it first thins out, or effaces, and then begins to open, or dilate. The cervix has to open to about 10 centimeters before birth can take place. For a first baby the cervix may not change much prior to labor. It is more usual to have some effacement and dilation of a few centimeters prior to labor in subsequent pregnancies.

Labor and Delivery

You've probably completed a prepared-childbirth course, but if this is your first pregnancy, you really don't know what labor and delivery are going to be like. By now many women will have shared their experiences with you, especially the horror stories or the glorified easy events when pain was almost nonexistent and when, start to finish, labor and delivery only took an hour and a half. Forget the stories. For the vast majority of us labor and delivery are neither ghastly, horrifying experiences nor complete pleasure every step of the way.

What, then, should you expect? The onset of labor is signaled by true contractions. Unlike Braxton-Hicks contractions, those of real labor are regular and travel from back to front. Some women experience them almost entirely abdominally and others almost exclusively in the back. Usually they start 15 to 20 minutes apart and last about half a minute. Each contraction builds in intensity, reaches a peak, and then dissipates rather quickly. The contractions may at first resemble menstrual cramps. They are progressive: as time passes, they get closer together, last longer, and become stronger. Unlike the Braxton-Hicks contractions, they do not go away with activity.

Labor begins under a variety of circumstances. You may be awakened in bed by contractions, or the first pains may come while you're doing the laundry or arguing a case in court. No doubt it's coincidental, but many of my friends have started labor at the end of a late evening out, particularly after eating hot, spicy foods. When I drove to the hospital at midnight with my husband after a Middle Eastern feast, I worried about the aroma of curries, chutneys, and wine on my labor-panting breath! I was also concerned about starting labor when both of us needed sleep; Leon solved this problem by promptly falling asleep on the only available stretcher in the maternity ward.

In about 10% of women the membranes rupture before the onset of labor; the amniotic sac has broken and a gush or steady trickle of waterlike fluid is expelled. It is usually painless; you might wonder if you've suddenly wet your pants. You may leave a puddle in the supermarket, but it's more likely to happen in bed. If it does occur, be sure to let your doctor know. Usually you are told to come to the hospital because labor is expected to begin quite soon. One woman reported rupture to her practitioner, who was on his way to an out-of-town medical convention. He erroneously told her that she wouldn't go into labor until his return several days later, and she didn't know enough to question this. Her baby was born that night, delivered by a doctor she'd never seen before. If labor does not start within 12 to 24 hours after the water has broken, and the baby is not preterm, labor will be induced. There's a good reason for this: the baby's chance of infection increases if your membranes are ruptured for more than 24 hours.

Another early sign of the onset of labor, occurring in 90% of women, is the passage of a pink/red-tinged plug of mucus often referred to as "show" or "bloody show." This plug, which has served as a stopper or barrier between the cervix and vagina, drops out as the cervix begins to thin and dilate. You don't feel it happen, but you'll probably notice the show. In most instances you'll begin labor within 48 hours.

First Stage of Labor

Labor is considered to have three stages, the first being the longest. During stage one, the contractions of the uterus progress in rate, intensity, and effectiveness until the cervix is totally dilated at 10 centimeters so the baby can pass through. With a first baby, the process usually takes 10 to 13 hours. Second and subsequent babies usually mean progressively shorter labors, but you can't count on it.

The first stage of labor has three phases: early, active, and transition. In the early phase, contractions begin and are usually infrequent and mild, although they may start strongly. During the active phase the contractions come at shorter and shorter intervals until they're only about two minutes apart, and they lengthen until each one lasts 50 to 60 seconds. At some point during this active phase—usually when the contractions are well established at five- or six-minute intervals—you'll notify your practitioner according to his or her instructions and proceed to your birth center or hospital. Once there, you'll complete the active phase of labor, by the end of which you'll be 8 centimeters dilated, and move into transition, during which the cervix will complete its dilation.

If your membranes did not rupture at the onset of labor, they will do so at some time during the first stage. Occasionally, to speed up labor, the attending physician will puncture the membranes before they burst spontaneously. You won't be allowed to eat during labor, because digestion shuts down for the duration, and you probably won't be allowed to drink either. Sour balls, lollipops, and ice chips are pleasant and permissible—bring some of the former with you, and locate a source of the latter at your birth center.

Transition is the most difficult phase of labor with which to cope. Contractions increase markedly in intensity, lasting for up to 90 seconds, or even more, and there's very little time in between them. You may feel nauseous or vomit now, which is another reason not to eat once labor pains begin. The pain and passage of time are getting to you; you begin to feel out of control and long for a rest break before going on. You may start to shiver uncontrollably and sweat heavily. You're likely to become irritable and snap at your partner, the doctor, the midwife, anyone who's handy. Any relaxation techniques you've learned can give you crucial assistance now, as can a labor coach. If you tense up during each contraction, you counteract the work the uterus is doing to open the cervix; you lengthen the labor and make it harder to get through. And if you're tense, you can't relax between contractions, when blood supply returns to the baby and the uterine muscle.

If labor does not proceed well, with weak or erratic uterine contractions, it may be augmented artificially. Oxytocin, a hormone that has a strong stimulating effect on the uterine muscles, is now produced synthetically; one common trade name is

Pitocin. Oxytocin is administered intravenously, by a "drip" or tube inserted into a vein in your arm. The flow can be adjusted up or down with a corresponding effect on the strength of contractions. Oxytocin is also used to induce labor—to start and maintain it when it doesn't happen spontaneously. Induction may be indicated if you are more than two weeks past your due date, if the placenta seems to be functioning poorly, or if continued pregnancy for any reason seems hazardous to the fetus. Naturally, the baby's ability to survive outside the womb must be evaluated carefully before beginning induction.

As you go through labor you will be periodically checked by a physician, nurse, or midwife, to see what progress the cervix is making in effacement and dilation. You may also be monitored electronically. A wide belt is attached to your belly; you can then see your baby's heartbeats and your contractions pictorially on a small TV-like screen or a printout. Or, after the membranes have ruptured and the cervix has dilated sufficiently, a spiral electrode may be attached to the baby's scalp. This is a brief but uncomfortable procedure. The internal monitor, too, depicts your baby's heartbeats. It's considered more precise and comprehensive than the external monitor.

Due to your age, there may be a tendency to follow your labor closely via this electronic fetal monitoring. This will hamper your ability to walk around and change position during labor, which may be vital to avoid the longer labor expected for an older woman. Few obstetricians would want to do without electronic fetal monitoring. If circumstances warrant, though, many practitioners will agree, or even plan routinely, to use it at intervals during labor. This leaves you relatively unrestrained while providing a sophisticated check on fetal well-being during contractions. A new method of monitoring labor called fetal telemetry is now being developed in which a monitoring device is inserted into the vagina like a tampon. It transmits signals without being connected to the readout machine and so permits complete mobility plus continuous monitoring.

You may find fetal monitoring invasive and uncomfortable, and it does statistically increase your already elevated chances of having a cesarean delivery. However, monitoring has saved the lives of many, many babies and has saved many others from being born with a lifelong handicap created by fetal distress during labor.

Questions of medication arise sometime during the first stage of labor. You may go all the way through without any, or you may choose one of several kinds of pain relief. It's best not to set down any hard and fast rules. Each circumstance is different. If your labor starts at midnight after a long, tiring day, you can't expect your stamina to be the same as if labor had started at 8 A.M. after a restful night. Your second labor may not be anything like your first; you may need medication this time although you didn't before, or the opposite may be true. In general, the medical community does not recommend much medication at the outset, because it might slow down labor and have a negative effect on the baby. Later in stage one, however, pain relief is more acceptable.

If you have an intravenous in place, medication can be administered through this tube. It will act on your entire body. Pain relievers can also be injected. Analgesics, such as Demerol, act on the central nervous system and provide quick relief. Unlike anesthesia, they do not block pain but dull the sensation of it. Because general anesthesia produces unconsciousness, it is seldom used in labor and delivery except for some cesarean sections. Regional anesthesia is administered through a needle placed in your lower back (epidural, caudal, or spinal block) or by injection in or around the birth canal (paracervical or pudendal block), numbing the lower part of your body. A regional block takes away the urge to push and often necessitates a forceps delivery, discussed below. Circumstances peculiar to your situation dictate what sort of pain-relieving medication would be best for you and what would harm your baby the least.

Second Stage of Labor (Delivery)

At the end of the first stage of labor, the cervix is fully dilated. During the second, or delivery, stage the baby moves through the birth canal and is delivered. The uterine contractions alone can propel the baby, but you can speed the process up a lot by consciously pushing along with the contractions. With your first baby, this stage is likely to last an hour or two; the time shrinks to half an hour or less for most later babies.

The onset of this second stage is heralded by an increasing desire to push. You may at first think you want to move your bowels, and you might, involuntarily. If you've had an enema, there isn't anything much to expel. You'll be advised not to push until you're fully dilated and will find it hard to remain relaxed without bearing down during contractions. The command, finally to go ahead and push, comes as a tremendous relief. The rhythm of labor changes as you participate in the contractions which, although stronger, are spaced somewhat farther apart. Photographs of laboring women show a contorted, grimacing face, but the expression is caused not so much by pain as by the overwhelming effort the mother is exerting. Pushing through each contraction may make the pain of contraction much less noticeable. Your total concentration is on pushing the baby to delivery. Everyone in the labor room seems to be participating now. Coach, nurses, and practitioner cluster around and help you hold your preferred position during each push. In between contractions you will relax and regroup for the next effort; you may even nod off.

As the uterus contracts and you push, the baby is pressed against the pelvic floor. Often the baby's scalp can be seen at the vaginal opening. The labor-room group seems to turn into a cheering squad—"Come on! Another good push! There's the head!" Everyone else present has a good view; if you want to see what's happening, you have to watch it in mirrors, which are usually set up or available wherever you're delivering but are convex and hard to see into clearly. It really irked my friend Kate that she was going through all this strain, effort, and pain and everyone except her got to see the baby's head crowning. "John! Come look at this!" the midwife cried to the father when the head first showed. Kate wanted to run down and look herself. It was her turn to feel left out.

As the baby's head passes through the pelvic opening, it rotates so it is almost always facing the mother's spine. You'll feel tremendous pressure as it begins to push against and stretch the vaginal opening. At this point your practitioner may perform an episiotomy, in which a small cut is made in the skin and muscle just behind the vagina called the perineum, to prevent any possible tearing.

After a few more contractions, the baby's head finally emerges—first the top, then the forehead, face, and neck. Your birth attendant will check to be sure the umbilical cord isn't wound around the baby's neck and will remove it if it is; the baby's nose and mouth will be cleared. Your baby may take its first breath and utter its first cry now, before it fully emerges. With your next contractions the shoulders will appear, followed by the rest of the body. Your practitioner may be able to slow things down a bit after the shoulders are out so you can sit up and watch the infant emerge fully.

If the second stage of labor lasts much more than two hours, your practitioner may decide to use forceps to help the baby's delivery. The instrument fits around the baby's head and can be used to ease the baby along as well as to rotate the baby's head and protect the soft skull of a premature infant. If forceps are applied, you may be given anesthesia. In some cases of delayed or complicated delivery, a vacuum suction device will be substituted for forceps.

As you alternately push and pant, particularly as the head emerges, you'll feel as though all of your insides are coming out—they're not, just the baby. The baby's umbilical cord is clamped and cut and her or his cry, skin color, reflexes, respiration, and heart rate are checked, while you lie there afterward, euphoric and utterly fatigued. Based on these readings, the baby is accorded an Apgar score of 0 to 10; most infants rate 7 or better. The baby will be handed to you and your partner at some point before, during, or after all this. Many fathers are now allowed to cut the umbilical cord, and your baby can be put to the breast immediately, even before the cord is cut.

Third Stage of Labor

The third stage occurs quickly and usually with little effort. After another mild contraction or two, the placenta separates from the wall of the uterus and is delivered. Sometimes it's helped along by a slight push on your abdomen from one of the delivery-room personnel. Occasionally the placenta is not expelled spontaneously and is then removed by hand under general or regional anesthesia. Your practitioner will examine the placenta to be sure none remains in the uterus. If you had an episiotomy, it will be repaired now, with a little local anesthetic and several stitches. Your uterus will continue to contract mildly as it reduces itself back toward its prepregnant size. Nursing your baby will stimulate these contractions.

You've exerted yourself to the limit, and you've delivered your baby. Suddenly that enormous swollen belly is gone and you can feel your hip bones for the first time in months. You feel surprisingly good, mentally and physically, but as the excitement ebbs you begin to drowse off. You may also get the shakes again; a warm blanket can feel heavenly. Your partner, too, has expended a lot of energy and can feel the fatigue underlying his exhilaration.

Depending on your birth setting and method, you'll be taken to a recovery room or your postbirth hospital room or you'll stay in the room in which you labored and delivered. Your baby may stay with you or be taken to a nursery; your partner may room in with you or have to leave after several hours. You don't know which to do first: sleep (you keep nodding off), eat (you're ravenous), or call all your friends and relatives. There's plenty of time for it all. Lie back and be proud of what you've accomplished. Congratulations!

There are, of course, many variations of labor. It is a natural process, but it's also intricate. Complications more common in older mothers that might arise are discussed in the following chapter. There are also a number of different approaches to managing labor and delivery. The options open to you are considered in Chapter 8. The postpartum weeks introduce new physical and psychological factors, which are discussed in Chapter 11.

CHAPTER 6

PROBLEMS IN PREGNANCY

Being over 35 and pregnant in the 1980's is exhilarating. You're doing something that wasn't considered advisable 10 or 20 years ago. Then, you would in almost all cases have been classified as "high risk" and simply told not to get pregnant. Today, problem pregnancies and possible problem pregnancies can be accurately identified. Problems diagnosed can be treated.

Advances in medical techniques together with increased knowledge about nutrition and fitness enable you to be treated in nearly the same way as your 30– or 25-year-old pregnant counterpart. "Nearly," because there are still some risks associated with pregnancy that are somewhat more likely to be experienced by the over-35 woman, and your practitioner will be somewhat more alert to their possibility.

You and your partner may be worried about your over–35 pregnancy, or you might be quite unconcerned about age-related factor, or perhaps you might start off unworried and become concerned only after listening to friends, relatives, and acquaintances express their hazy conceptions about the risks of older childbearing. The best way to deal with anyone's concerns, including your own, is to be informed. This chapter discusses those risks that women over 35 may be more likely to face than younger women, and it will describe ways to avoid or deal with those complications.

Genetics

The most familiar risk of pregnancy for an older woman is the possibility of conceiving a child with a chromosomal abnormality, specifically Down's syndrome. Each cell in your body has 23 pairs of chromosomes which in turn contain strands of paired genes. The egg and the sperm each contain only 23 single chromosomes; they unite at conception to form 23 pairs. Sometimes, rarely, there is a missing chromosome, an extra chromosome, or a damaged chromosome. As the cells in the developing embryo, then fetus, divide and multiply, each one reproduces the chromosomal abnormality. Since each chromosome contains so many genes, each of which affects some particular aspect of a baby's development, a chromosomal imbalance can result in multiple defects.

Unfortunately, chromosomal disorders become more likely as a woman ages. These risks do not change as medical technology advances; chromosomal abnormalities are not yet an avoidable hazard. The charts that follow show the age-related increase found in two comprehensive studies of live births. (Anencephaly and spina bifida, neural tube defects, are described in the section on AFP testing in Chapter 4.)

Down's syndrome, in which an extra chromosome is present, figures as the most common of these chromosomal abnormalities. A child born with Down's will be mentally retarded—mildly or severely—and likely to have other health problems, such as a heart defect and greater susceptibility to respiratory infections. Down's also produces a rather flat face and eyes that appear slightly slanted, giving an Oriental appearance; because of this, Down's used to be called mongolism, a person so affected, a mongoloid. A baby conceived with Down's or other serious chromosomal abnormalities has an increased risk of dying in the uterus or soon after birth. Those who do survive birth have a significantly reduced life expectancy after the age of 40.

While younger women give birth to the greatest number of Down's children because they have the greatest number of babies, an older woman has a greater chance than a younger one of conceiving a child with Down's syndrome. The following charts show the rising degree of risk as a woman ages.

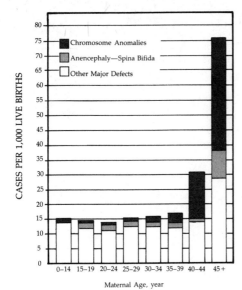

Incidence of selected major birth defects by maternal age, metropolitan Atlanta, 1968 to 1975.

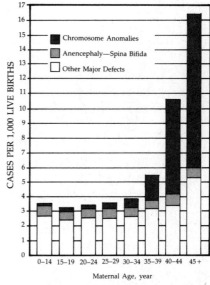

Incidence of selected major birth defects by maternal age, National Center for Health Statistics, 1973 to 1975.

[Source: Marshall F. Goldberg, Larry D. Edmonds, and Godfrey P. Oakley, "Reducing Birth Defect Risk in Advanced Maternal Age," reprinted by permission of the authors and *JAMA* (Journal of the American Medical Association), 242:21 (November 23, 1979), p. 2293.] Copyright 1979, American Medical Association.

Relationship of Down's Syndrome to Maternal Age

Mother's Age	Incidence of Down's Syndrome
under 30	less than 1 in 1,000
30	1 in 900
35	1 in 400
36	1 in 300
37	1 in 230
38	1 in 180
39	1 in 135
40	1 in 105
42	1 in 60
44	1 in 35
46	1 in 20
48	1 in 12

[Source: National Institute of Child Health and Human Development, National Institutes of Health, June 1982.]

Opinion and evidence are mixed as to whether congenital abnormalities and genetic defects not involving entire chromosomes are any more likely for babies of older mothers. Some studies have found a somewhat higher incidence of malformations such as polydactyly (extra fingers or toes) and cleft lip and palate—often easily correctible conditions—and spina bifida and heart defects. Yet other studies contradict this and conclude that increased risk of malformation is, if anything, extremely small. For example, the birth defect chart based on the Atlanta study shows no consistent increase in neural tube defects related to age and no statistically significant increase in other major defects until after age 44.

Why do chromosomal abnormalities increase as a woman gets older? It's not known for certain, but several factors have been implicated, among which egg age may be the most important. Since a woman is born with all the eggs she'll ever have, the egg that gets fertilized to produce your child is as old as you are. It is thought that aging of the eggs and ovaries may lead to egg degeneration. In addition to simply aging, an older woman's eggs have had more years of exposure to toxins: radiation (natural and manufactured), pollutants, drugs. This may in turn affect the chromosomal makeup of the eggs. Or aging ovaries may release immature or overmature eggs which, again, may therefore be chromosomally defective. These theories, unfortunately, remain hypothetical.

The role of the father's age is not known, either. Sperm do not age as eggs do; sperm are produced continuously and have a short life span. Nevertheless, a man's reproductive system and body age, and he too accumulates exposure to environmental hazards. A growing body of evidence suggests that older men, especially those over 45, are more likely to produce children with birth defects. For example, a 10-year Norwegian examination of birth records, reported in the *Journal of Medical Genetics* (February 1981), found a "modestly increased" risk of Down's syndrome associated with fathers over 50, independent of any maternal age effect. Ernest B. Hook of New York State's Birth Defects Institute, the author of many Down's syndrome studies, stated in the September 1981 issue of *Obstetrics and Gynecology* that data linking paternal age and Down's is suggestive but not conclusive; there is as yet no concrete proof that a father's age affects the likelihood of chromosomal abnormalities in his children. Hook holds to that conclusion today. Certain malformations caused by gene mutations rather than chromosome irregularities do, however, seem to be more common in children of older fathers although they are still rare. Much more research needs to be done to accumulate knowledge in this area before any conclusions can be reached.

Fortunately, doctors are capable of diagnosing Down's syndrome and a number of other chromosomal abnormalities by amniocentesis—the testing of the amniotic fluid and the fetal cells found in it—which was described in Chapter 4. The capability of diagnosing Down's and other chromosomal defects in an unborn child plus the availability of abortion has transformed childbearing for women over 35. The major risk, one that is untreatable, can be identified and then, if a couple so chooses, nullified through abortion.

A study of 3,000 amniocenteses found the following incidence of both Down's syndrome and all chromosomal abnormalities in the second trimester of pregnancy.

Maternal Age	Down's Syndrome	All Chromosomal Abnormalities
35–36	1/143	1/66
37–38	1/100	1/54
39–40	1/45	1/35
41–42	1/41	1/31
43–44	1/18	1/10

[Source: M. Golbus et al., "Prenatal Genetic Diagnosis in 3000 Amniocenteses," excerpted by permission of *The New England Journal of Medicine*, 300:157 (January 23, 1979).]

A Japanese analysis published in *Obstetrics and Gynecology* (November 1978) found chromosomal abnormalities in one out of four aborted embryos of women 45 to 49. These rates are much higher than those for live births shown in the birth-defect and Down's syndrome charts. Perhaps one third of chromosomally defective fetuses detected early in the second trimester will die spontaneously; the rest of the difference between numbers of diagnosed abnormalities and live births is accounted for by induced abortion.

Of course, not all couples will be willing to terminate a pregnancy. But knowing that it's possible gives an over-35 couple the freedom to conceive without subjecting themselves to a significantly increased possibility of having to care for a severely handicapped child. Goldberg and his coauthors, who drew up the birth-defect charts, estimated that, given amniocentesis and a willingness to abort, the odds of a woman between 35 and 45 having a baby with severe birth defects are the same as the odds for younger women. The risk reduction possible, these researchers report, is up to 46% for women 35 to 39 and 68% for women 40 and over.

Amniocentesis can even avert abortions. Some couples at risk (for any reason, not just age) of conceiving a child with birth defects may choose to abort a pregnancy unless a test can show that the fetus appears to be normal. Not every abnormality is a cause for abortion, however, and different parents will react differently to the same problem. Sometimes amniocentesis reveals a chromosomal abnormality whose effects or degree of severity cannot be predicted, requiring the most difficult decisions from prospective parents.

The major problem with amniocentesis is that you're 20

weeks pregnant by the time you get the results. You've started your second trimester, and it's certainly not the optimal time, physically or psychologically, to have an abortion. New technology may change this, specifically, a process called chorionic villus sampling, or chorion villus biopsy, in which a tiny bit of the chorion, part of the developing placenta, is extracted. Chorion villus sampling can be done in the sixth to eighth week of pregnancy. Many more cells are present in the sample than in amniotic fluid, and they are rapidly dividing, so readable results of genetic testing are available within a few days. However, chorionic villus sampling is still considered semi-experimental. Only a limited number of centers are equipped to do the testing, and questions remain as to accuracy and risks, specifically of spontaneous abortion. At Jefferson Hospital in Philadelphia, one of the few centers where a number of chorion villus samplings have been performed, the miscarriage rate following the procedure is quoted as 1.5% to 2%; worldwide, it's estimated at 3% to 5%. Incorrect results can be reported if, for example, maternal rather than fetal cells are mistakenly tested. Because the safety and accuracy rates have not been firmly established, the National Institutes of Health are now embarking on an evaluation of chorionic villus sampling at seven centers nationwide. Limitations on availability and scientific evaluation mean that amniocentesis remains the method of choice to test for genetic defects in utero. Nevertheless, Dr. Delphine Bartosik, director of reproductive endocrinology at Hahnemann University Hospital, says of chorionic villus sampling, "I'm thoroughly certain that over a period of time, it's going to almost completely replace amniocentesis."

Other tests now being developed include one called ATA which stands, logically enough, for Alternative to Amniocentesis. This procedure, which is still also very experimental, involves a blood test early in pregnancy. It was developed by microbiologists at Michigan State University.

Another still-experimental method of diagnosing birth defects is fetoscopy. In this procedure, a tiny lighted tube and lens are inserted through the abdomen into the amniotic sac. The doctor can actually see the fetus and any visible abnormalities. Fetoscopy also allows a doctor to take very small samples of fetal blood and skin for testing. Like chorionic villus sampling, fetoscopy will remain experimental and rarely used until its accompanying complication rate, including spontaneous abortion, is substantially reduced.

On the horizon are startling new methods of treating, not just diagnosing, genetic defects and congenital abnormalities. Microsurgical and prenatal diagnostic techniques have combined to make surgery inside the uterus, on the fetus itself, possible. It is of course very risky and rarely resorted to because it's so difficult to judge the severity of the fetal problem and so likely to result in spontaneous abortion. "There are no surgical miracles in the womb," says bioethicist Dr. John C. Fletcher of the National Institutes of Health (*Medical World News*, December 10, 1984), but surgery in utero will become more common as knowledge increases and methods are improved. Genetic engineering and genetic therapy are also possibilities, whereby genetic defects are diagnosed and then treated or corrected in utero via injections of missing genetic material. Future developments in these areas are certain to be dramatic. For now, however, "Genetic engineering is still fantasy," Dr. Bartosik states.

Chronic and Gestational Conditions

Chronic Disease

Besides the risk of chromosomal abnormalities, women over 35 are more likely than younger women to have a chronic health problem that could affect the pregnancy. The older you are, the more possible it is that you have developed a condition such as heart or kidney disease, respiratory disorders, diabetes, and thyroid problems. It can be tricky to treat these conditions in a way that is compatible with pregnancy, and the illnesses themselves can complicate the pregnancy considerably. You will require the careful attention of your practitioner and perhaps referral to a specialist or a high-risk clinic. But 35 is really quite young to have developed any of these problems; the odds are that you haven't, in which case an entire category of risk is wiped out.

Fibroids

There are a number of reproductive system disorders that you are prone to as you get older, particularly fibroid tumors, or benign growths, in the uterus. These conditions are discussed in Chapter 2 because they affect fertility more than pregnancy. But fibroid tumors may interfere with your ability to carry a baby to term, causing miscarriage or preterm labor. They may also make labor more difficult. Once you've become pregnant, there's not much you can do about fibroids; if they're small enough, they're not likely to cause a problem. Even when they're serious, full-term pregnancy can be achieved. This was the case with Marcia, who had five miscarriages caused by fibroids, but twice an ovum found a rare spot within the uterus to implant successfully. Her two healthy babies were born when she was 34 and 39.

High Blood Pressure, Pre-eclampsia, and Toxemia

One medical condition that is found more often in women over 35 (pregnant or not) than in younger women is high blood pressure, or hypertension. This condition can seriously complicate pregnancy. High blood pressure means your arteries are compressing or constricting too much as the heart pumps blood through them. Since your blood volume expands dramatically during pregnancy, any tendency you may have toward hypertension is likely to be aggravated now. If your blood pressure is high before you become pregnant, or rises in the early weeks of pregnancy, you're said to have "chronic" or "essential" hypertension—not pregnancy-induced. Your blood pressure may also rise during pregnancy; this is called "gestational" hypertension.

High blood pressure is serious because it interferes with the critical flow of oxygen and nutrients to the fetus. To treat it, your practitioner will prescribe plenty of bed rest and extra attention to nutrition. You may have to drop strenuous exercise of any kind and watch your salt intake. You'll also need more frequent checkups than once a month, to monitor both your blood pressure and any swelling or sudden weight gain.

These last two symptoms can be a sign that your high blood pressure is leading to a serious complication of pregnancy called pre-eclampsia, in which hypertension couples with excessive fluid retention and loss of protein through the urine. This condition in turn can lead to eclampsia, or toxemia, in which convulsions accompany the pre-eclampsia. While toxemia is life-threatening to both mother and fetus, well-nourished women who receive attentive prenatal care rarely develop it, and it's actually more common among younger mothers. Pre-eclampsia occurs more often than toxemia. While some studies report that pre-eclampsia occurs more often in women over 35 than in younger expectant mothers, others question this conclusion. Pre-eclampsia can be mild or severe. The most serious cases can reduce placental circulation and protein availability enough to threaten the life of the fetus. Treatment is the same as for simple hypertension but may be more comprehensive: hospitalization may be necessary, plus frequent evaluation of weight, kidney function, and blood pressure. If your pre-eclampsia is severe, your doctor may decide to induce delivery early—usually at 35 weeks or so—rather than have you continue the pregnancy.

Gestational Diabetes

Another condition more common in over-35 pregnant women than in their younger counterparts is gestational diabetes—diabetes that develops during pregnancy. Diabetes is a disorder in which the body fails to produce enough, or becomes resistant to the available, insulin—a hormone that regulates the conversion of sugar to energy and the storing of sugar for future energy needs. To replace this fuel, the body breaks down stored fat and releases acids, which in turn upsets the body's chemical balance and threatens many organs. During pregnancy, the developing fetus depletes your glucose supply and places other strains on your metabolism, increasing your risk of developing diabetes now. To monitor for this risk, your urine sample will be checked at each prenatal visit for the presence of glucose. Your blood-sugar level will also be checked once or twice during your pregnancy.

You'll probably be able to control gestational diabetes under your doctor's guidance by a diet that maintains your blood sugar at normal or nearly normal levels. Sometimes, however, insulin injections may be needed. The important thing is to monitor and regulate the condition, because uncontrolled, it greatly increases the risks of stillbirth and birth defects, especially late in pregnancy, due to placental insufficiency. Known diabetics should optimize control of blood-sugar levels before conceiving, to lower the risk of birth defects during early fetal development. While babies born to diabetic women are at risk for a number of problems immediately after birth, such as respiratory difficulties, low blood sugar, and jaundice, good neonatal care can usually treat them successfully.

Complications of Pregnancy, Labor, and Delivery

Placental Problems

Two placental problems are more likely to be experienced by the over-35 pregnant woman than by younger women. One, called placenta previa, occurs when the placenta is implanted low in the uterus, close to or over the opening of the cervix. During the third trimester the cervix softens and may start to dilate. If the placenta is situated over the cervix when this happens, it may tear; you will then be likely to experience bleeding. This bleeding may be intermittent, continuous, or gushing, but is usually painless. If you have had ultrasound at an earlier point in pregnancy, it is very likely that the placement of your placenta will be known. If you've got placenta previa and begin to bleed, you will be admitted to the hospital and carefully evaluated. If neither you nor your baby is in distress, delivery will be postponed until week 36 to allow time for the baby to mature, helped by bed rest and blood replacement as necessary. You may even be given a drug to help the baby's lungs develop faster. Occasionally, a vaginal delivery can be done, if the placenta blocks only part of the cervix. In most cases of placenta previa, however, doctors find it necessary to perform a cesarean section. Should you have this complication, state-of-the-art obstetrics has greatly improved the likelihood of a good outcome for you and your baby.

The other placental problem somewhat more prevalent in over-35 mothers than in younger ones is abruptio placenta, or premature separation of the placenta from the uterus. The separation may be partial or complete. There may be painless vaginal bleeding, or severe contractions and no external bleeding. The condition can be diagnosed by ultrasound. The threat to the baby is a reduction or termination of its oxygen/nutrient supply. The threat to you is blood loss and shock. The most severe cases are extremely serious emergencies for both mother and child; fortunately, they are also rare. The more serious abruptions frequently require cesarean sections.

The table below charts the age-related incidence of these two placental problems found in an analysis of over 44,000 pregnancies.

Condition	Maternal Age (year)				
	17–19	20–30	31–34	35–39	40–50
Placenta previa (cases per 1000 births)	3	6	10	11	24
Abruptio placenta (cases per 1000 births)	13	20	27	25	32

[Source: Richard L. Naeye, M.D., "Maternal Age, Obstetric Complications, and the Outcome of Pregnancy," reprinted with permission from the author and The American College of Obstetricians and Gynecologists, *Obstetrics and Gynecology,* 61:2 (February 1983), p. 213.]

While both conditions do occur more often with age, you are unlikely to have either of them. However, if you have bleeding and/or severe cramping during your pregnancy, you should call your practitioner and get yourself to a hospital.

Abnormal Presentation

If you're over 35 you're also at higher risk for an abnormal presentation of the baby. Normally, during the last month of pregnancy, the baby settles head down into your pelvis; during delivery the baby exits head first. In about 1 out of 20 cases, however, the baby "presents" something other than his or her head. In most instances of abnormal presentation the baby emerges in the breech, or bottom first (buttocks or legs), position. This can make a vaginal delivery questionable, as there is a risk of the baby's head being caught in the pelvis, thereby cutting off the oxygen supply.

To avoid this danger, your obstetrician may try turning the baby in the uterus at 37 weeks. At that stage of gestation, a baby not already in the head-down position is unlikely to turn into it spontaneously. Also, the pressure exerted on the uterus during the turning may cause the membranes to rupture, making delivery necessary; at 37 weeks, the baby is term, so birth should pose no threat.

If turning doesn't work or is not an option in your case, the size of the baby's head and your pelvis will be carefully evaluated to see if vaginal delivery, possible for some breech births, is feasible for you. Forceps will probably be used to protect the baby's head, which means also you'll probably have an epidural. Because many obstetricians take a very cautious approach toward over-35 women in labor, and because such women may have somewhat longer labors, doctors often advise a cesarean delivery for breech positions. This is especially true if the baby is premature and so judged less able to withstand the stress of labor and delivery successfully.

Multiple Pregnancy

Multiple births are another "risk" you face as an older prospective mother. Multiple conception occurs when a fertilized egg divides or when more than one egg is fertilized. The peak age for twinning is 37. The odds overall are highest between 35 and 39. Your chances are further increased if you are taking a fertility drug, if you've had several other children (especially twins), or if your mother has a fraternal twin.

Carrying twins is tricky because complications are more frequent. Half of all twins are born prematurely, and they are likely to be small for their gestational age, both of which factors threaten their survival in the weeks after birth. Twins are also at increased risk of stillbirth and are somewhat more likely to have congenital malformations. Genetic defects are no more common but may be harder to detect because of the difficulty of testing two fetuses. Abnormal presentation for delivery, while still not usual, is more likely for twins. In a multiple pregnancy, you stand a greater chance of pre-eclampsia or toxemia, gestational hypertension, and gestational diabetes.

How can you tell if yours is a multiple pregnancy? Your weight will increase and your abdomen will expand much faster than normally. Your practitioner will check the height of your uterus and your hormone levels. When twins are suspected, your practitioner will try to detect multiple heartbeats. Ultrasound again provides the tool to make a positive diagnosis.

Because of the potential complications when you're carrying more than one child, attention to your overall health is even more important than ever. Good nutrition is crucial to meet the increased demands of the extra baby or babies. Many of the minor complaints of pregnancy, such as breathlessness, heartburn, and swelling, will be aggravated. You'll need extra rest and no strenuous exercise. You'll be carefully monitored by your practitioner, especially since premature labor is so likely.

Your obstetrician's preference for delivery will depend on the position, age, and size of the babies, as well as the progress of labor. However, the overstretched uterus may not contract strongly enough during labor and so, to counteract this problem, an intravenous contraction-augmenting medication may be administered. With improved prenatal diagnosis and care (especially methods to delay preterm labor), improved obstetrical techniques, and today's neonatal treatment, the prognosis for multiple births is currently very good.

Prolonged Labor

You may be subjected to a longer and more complicated labor than younger women. This is particularly true in the case of first delivery. The uterus does lose some elasticity with age, which can prolong labor but not necessarily complicate it. On the other hand, if you're physically fit and have good muscle tone, a somewhat less elastic uterus may not affect delivery. Also, if you are fortunate enough to remain free from medical complications and in good health, age as such should not cause a more difficult labor and delivery. Prepared childbirth, too, helps avoid or lessen extended labor. But take note, several nurses, childbirth instructors, and obstetricians I spoke with emphasized the importance for the older mother of walking and moving around during labor to speed things along.

Cesarean Delivery

Delivery by cesarean section unquestionably occurs more often for women over 35 than for younger mothers. In 1981 the c-section rate in the United States was 13.2% for women under 20, rising to 17.7% for mothers 20 to 29, and peaking at 24.4% for women 35 and over. That's just about one out of every four births to older mothers.

Many of the complications mentioned earlier in this chapter may necessitate a cesarean section, such as large uterine tumors, severe hypertension, diabetes, and placental abnormalities. Abdominal delivery is also indicated if you have an active herpes infection, to protect the baby from contact with the virus. Unfortunately, a prior cesarean may also be an indication for subsequent cesareans. Repeat c-sections account for approximately 30% of the increase in abdominal deliveries.

A cesarean delivery requires anesthesia because it involves

an incision in the abdomen and uterus so the baby can be lifted out. Planned c-sections can usually be done with regional anesthesia. A needle with numbing medication is inserted into the area surrounding the spinal nerves so that you do not feel the lower part of your body; you can then be awake for the birth of your baby, although your view of the actual operation is blocked. If an emergency c-section is needed, general rather than regional anesthesia may be the best choice. In this case, you'll be out cold during the operation.

The incision is usually low and horizontal—the "bikini cut"; sometimes a long vertical cut is necessary. The low incision results in a less noticeable scar and also permits a subsequent vaginal delivery if the reason for the cesarean does not repeat itself. The vertical incision has a greater risk of rupturing during a subsequent labor, which is why "once a cesarean, always a cesarean" was an obstetric rule until recently. Your doctor may still adhere to it. Discuss the situation before you go into labor.

A good obstetrician can get a baby out with a c-section in a few minutes, literally, if either baby or mother are in serious trouble. This is one important argument in favor of hospital delivery. Fathers are usually now allowed to be present at cesarean births; you'll appreciate some support. Ask ahead of time to be sure there's no last-minute unwanted shuttling off of Dad to the waiting room. A c-section forces you to be hospitalized approximately five to seven days instead of the more usual three or less. Recovery will be slower than with vaginal delivery; you'll have some abdominal pain and gas for a few days, and your return to a normal routine of exercise and activity will be delayed. You will also find it harder to get back to your prepregnant shape.

Cesarean delivery has its pros and cons. On the one hand, the procedure saves fetal and maternal lives in cases where vaginal delivery just isn't possible or will take longer than the baby can survive. And in many cases, it allows you to skip the pain of labor. On the other hand, a cesarean is major surgery, and as such, carries risk, especially of maternal infection or clotting and depressed fetal reactions. Cesarean babies have lower Apgar scores than vaginally delivered babies and also experience a high incidence of respiratory distress syndrome, a serious breathing disorder.

Undergoing a c-section when you and your partner had planned a "natural" vaginal delivery can be very distressing. You may feel guilty and depressed, and deprived of the opportunity to participate actively in the birth. Bonding between parents and baby becomes more difficult, especially if the infant is whisked away to the nursery for 24 hours of observation and you're groggy from the anesthetic. The after-surgery pain and gas and the difficulty you'll have getting around for the first few days don't help psychologically, either. Nevertheless, there's tremendous exhilaration due to the fact that your baby has been born successfully. And if the survival of either of you would have been questionable without cesarean delivery, you'll feel nothing but gratitude for the procedure.

If you are going to need a cesarean, it's nice to know it ahead of time, although this isn't always possible. First, you and your partner can get mentally geared up for it and get all your questions formulated and answered. Second, you can plan the baby's time and place of birth, making specific work and childcare arrangements. Not only is this convenient for you, but also it's reassuring to any children you already have; Mommy doesn't just suddenly rush off and disappear on a moment's notice.

Considerable debate and controversy in obstetric and lay circles surrounds the rapidly rising percentage of cesarean deliveries in the United States. The August 1983 edition of the *American Journal of Public Health* reported that c-sections accounted for 5.5% of all deliveries in 1970 and shot up to 17.9% in 1981. This figure continues to rise. Why? The main reason is identification of dystocia (the unsatisfactory progression of labor, usually due to inefficient uterine contractions) and its management by abdominal delivery rather than by alternative methods such as oxytocin stimulation. Advances in fetal and neonatal care have a lot to do with it, too. Electronic fetal monitoring can identify fetal distress, and an endangered baby can often be better cared for in today's intensive-care nurseries than in the womb. While the operation is more risky for a mother than vaginal delivery, it's still considered very safe. Cesarean section is also preferred over high forceps delivery, in which the forceps are inserted into the upper birth canal. Doctors can be sued if a vaginal delivery results in a dead or handicapped infant. The family of a retarded six-year-old New York boy who suffered brain damage at birth sued the hospital where delivery took place for failing to perform a cesarean section as soon as monitoring disclosed abnormal fetal respiratory responses, indicating insufficient oxygen supply to the baby. While refusing to concede negligence, the hospital settled the suit in July 1984 for $11 million. For fear of a similar lawsuit, doctors may perform a cesarean in a moot case. An editorial in the *Journal of the American Medical Association* on December 21, 1984, commenting on the high rate of cesarean deliveries, declared, "Physician malpractice risk following poor outcome [of vaginal delivery in breech presentation] may be unsurmountable."

Doctors tend to be most conservative when faced with an older mother, especially a first-time one. There may be a sense that the baby is "premium"—that because of your age, you may not be able to replace this child, so any and all available measures should be taken to preserve it. Many doctors—and nurses, too, in a trickle-down effect—appear to have a higher anxiety level about the progress of an older woman's labor, although midwives don't seem to share this fear. Any signs of fetal distress or lengthy labor may prompt a call for cesarean delivery.

An illustration of this syndrome is Marty's experience during her first delivery at age 35. Her membranes ruptured, but she did not go into labor for more than 24 hours. Her obstetrician advised her to stay out of the hospital during that day-long period to avoid having a cesarean section urged on her. When Marty did enter the hospital, her labor progressed somewhat slowly. Her obstetrician, no longer "on call," came to the hospital anyway, and urged his partner, now the attending physician, to give Marty more time to labor as the partner several times decided a cesarean had become necessary in view of the length of labor and Marty's age. Thanks to the first obstetrician's intervention, Marty had a successful vaginal delivery.

Critics say that in many instances when cesareans are used, such as what almost happened to Marty, vaginal delivery would have been feasible. Fetal distress revealed by electronic fetal monitoring may be within the normal limits of labor stress and not an indication that a c-section is required. Although some doctors perform cesareans for all breech births, some breech presentations do permit vaginal delivery. Apparent disproportion between the size of the baby's head and the mother's pelvis does not always prevent vaginal delivery, either. Repeat cesareans are under fire, too. Many medical centers are now allowing women with previous cesareans to go into labor, with remarkable safety and success. A sampling of three medical journal articles on the outcomes of these "trials of labor" finds 67%, 79%, and 89% of mothers studied delivering vaginally after a prior c-section.

Cynics even suggest that doctors prefer cesareans because they can charge more for the surgery and can schedule their deliveries on a 9-to-5 basis! While the National Institutes of Health find no evidence to support those cynics, they have stated that the rising rate of cesarean delivery is "a matter of concern" and have concluded that the trend can be stopped and perhaps even reversed without preventing advances in maternal and fetal health. This conclusion is supported by a comparison of cesarean delivery rates in the United States in 1978 with the rates in Dublin, Ireland, in 1980, reported in *Obstetrics and Gynecology* (January 1983). Active management of labor, especially augmentation with oxytocin as discussed in the previous chapter, was found to be the major cause of the difference between the 4.8% Irish cesarean rate and the 15.2% U.S. rate; there was a steady drop in infant deaths at or close to birth during a 15-year period in Dublin although the percentage of cesarean deliveries remained unchanged.

Because a cesarean may become necessary for you or may be recommended by your practitioner, you and your partner should inform yourselves thoroughly about the procedure. You might want to ask your doctor how often he or she uses cesarean delivery. You might also want to check the c-section rate at the hospital where you'll deliver. Some hospitals have substantially higher rates than others. The August 1983 report in the *American Journal of Public Health* found the lowest percentages of cesarean deliveries at hospitals that were run by the U.S. government, had less than 100 beds, and were located in the North Central region of the country. Of women delivering at all hospitals, those who paid their own medical bills had the fewest cesareans.

If your hospital has a higher than average cesarean section

rate, find out why. There may be a standing protocol, for instance, that all first-time mothers with breech presentation be delivered abdominally. Although normally this would be at your obstetrician's discretion, she or he may agree with hospital policy. If your partner plans to be present during delivery, be sure your physician and the hospital are aware of this and have agreed to it ahead of time. Discuss what type of anesthetic you prefer, regional or general. Talk to others who have experienced cesarean birth, read some descriptions of it, and look at pictures. As with every other issue of pregnancy, the better informed and prepared you are, the better able you'll be to cope.

Fetal Loss

Over-35 women also experience a greater incidence of fetal loss. There are two types of fetal loss. One is miscarriage, defined as loss of a fetus before it could survive outside the womb, before the 26th or 28th week of gestation. The medical term for miscarriage is spontaneous abortion. The second type of loss is stillbirth, death of a fetus after about 28 weeks of gestation, when it was old enough to survive birth if it had been healthy.

A woman over 35 faces up to three times the possibility of miscarriage a woman in her 20's faces, although exact figures can't be given because very early miscarriage is often unrecognized when the pregnancy was unsuspected or unconfirmed. The most common reason for miscarriage is chromosomal abnormality. Nature aborts most grossly deformed fetuses. Since older women have a greater likelihood of conceiving a child with a chromosomal defect, it follows that their miscarriage risk is higher.

Stillbirth rates were examined in a recent study of childbearing women 30 to 39, which appeared in the *Journal of the American Medical Association* on December 14, 1984. Dr. Michele Forman and colleagues analyzed Swedish births from 1976 through 1980. Of women who had a previous live birth, the stillbirth rates were approximately 3 per 1,000 for ages 20 to 24, 4 per 1,000 for ages 30 to 34, and 6.5 per 1,000 for ages 35 to 39. Women never before pregnant experienced stillbirths at the rates of approximately 4.5 per 1,000 at ages 20 to 24, 6 per 1,000 at 30 to 34, and 8 per 1,000 at 35 to 39.

Whereas first trimester abortions do not seem to predispose you to a subsequent pregnancy loss, second trimester abortions do. Fortunately, experience is proving that today's suction method is far less likely to affect your ability to carry a subsequent pregnancy to term than the D & C technique (dilation and curettage) which was formerly used.

Prematurity

Early or preterm labor—labor occurring between the 20th and 37th weeks of pregnancy—is also more likely if you're over 35. Dr. Forman's figures from the Swedish study just mentioned confirm this, showing the following rates of prematurity per 1,000 cases:

Preterm Births (at or before 37 weeks)—Cases per Thousand

Maternal Age	No previous pregnancy	Previous miscarriage or induced abortion	Previous live birth
20–24	4.7	5.4	4
30–34	7	6.7	3.9
35–39	8	7.8	5.9

Source: Dr. Michele F. Forman, Division of Nutrition, Center for Disease Control, Atlanta, Georgia, as reported to the authors on the telephone in January, 1985.

Again, prematurity may be prompted by a complication or abnormal condition of pregnancy. Or it may occur with no prior warning. Prematurity is the single largest cause of newborn death. Fortunately, neonatology—the care of babies in the weeks just after birth—has developed very successful methods in the past 10 or 15 years. Babies as small as two pounds can survive. Current attention is focused on preventing preterm deliveries. The cervix can be checked periodically at prenatal visits for signs of "ripening"—lengthening, dilation, etc.—which may predict who will go into preterm labor. It's very important to recognize the signs of impending labor. They include cramps, abdominal pressure or tightness, low backache, and regularly spaced uterine contractions (four in 20 minutes, or eight in one hour) that you might only feel with your fingertips on your abdomen. Report these symptoms to your practitioner. If you are at risk for delivering preterm, you'll need extra rest and sleep, less exercise and activity, and as stress-free an environment as possible. Sexual intercourse may be banned to avoid uterine stimulation. If preterm labor seems imminent, you may be hospitalized and given labor-inhibiting drugs. You may also be given a medication to hasten maturation of the baby's lungs, a crucial factor in the infant's survival. Programs to delay preterm delivery are increasingly successful. Preventive measures include that familiar standby, good nutrition, plus no smoking.

Low Birth Weight

Some studies indicate that women over 35 are at greater risk of delivering babies with low birth weight. Dr. Forman's figures indicate that this is particularly true for women who have not had a previous live birth. A woman 35 to 39 in her first pregnancy was nearly 3 times more likely than a mother 20 to 24 to deliver a preterm, low birth weight baby, and 1½ times more likely to deliver a baby at term (38 weeks or later) with low birth weight. The rates were still a low 3.4 and 2.6 per thousand, respectively, for the older mothers, and they were even lower (1.8 and 1.2 per thousand) for the women 35 to 39 with a previous successful pregnancy.

Low birth weight is a condition independent of prematurity. A baby may be born at or close to term, but weigh less than expected for the length of its gestation. An infant weighing under 5½ pounds at birth may be classified preterm, small for its gestational age, or both. Low birth weight, like prematurity, is a serious threat to an infant's survival. An extra pound or two can make a crucial difference, especially if the baby has been born preterm and has to struggle through the first few days or weeks with organs and systems not yet fully mature. It can take several years for low-birth-weight children to catch up physically and intellectually with their peers.

Low birth weight is closely linked to socioeconomic status. Inadequate income leads to poor nutrition and, often, inadequate prenatal care. Insufficient fetal growth results. The incidence of first babies with low birth weight has decreased most for U.S. women in their 30's, a group that is composed, on the whole, of women more educated and financially better off than their younger counterparts. Not taking into account any medical complications, you should be able to avoid birth-weight problems with a nutritious diet, no smoking, and regular prenatal checkups.

Maternal Age and Risks: Conclusions

Many studies have been conducted on pregnancy in women aged 35 and over. All do find some increase in maternal and fetal complications. However, time and again the same basic conclusion is reached: If a woman is in good health, with no chronic disease, she may expect a successful pregnancy outcome whether she is in her late 30's, mid 20's, or early 40's, if amniocentesis is used to screen for chromosomal abnormalities and certain other defects. The increasing number of women over 35 giving birth demonstrates that pregnancy over 35 is not necessarily a hazardous proposition.

Should the Supreme Court or a constitutional amendment once again outlaw abortion, however, this conclusion would be gravely compromised. Women between 35 and 39 have an abortion rate 20% higher than that of the general population, while the rate for women over 40 is more than double the overall national figure. The results of amniocentesis do prompt a number of these abortions; however, many more are done for personal, nonmedical reasons. One group of researchers has estimated that "unselected abortion"—pregnancy termination not prompted by amniocentesis—averts five Down's syndrome births for every one or two averted by amniocentesis-prompted abortion (David A. Luthy and colleagues, *American Journal of Medical Genetics,* 1980). Legalized abortion, therefore, is a crucial factor in the good prognosis for over-35 pregnancy.

The risks that do exist for older women are borne most heavily by members of low socioeconomic groups and by less educated women, who tend also to be low on the socioeconomic scale. These women are more likely to have had many previous pregnancies—which increases all risk factors for mother and child—and are less likely to initiate and stick with adequate prenatal care. If the statistics for age-related complications were calculated without including women of low socioeconomic and educational levels, they would no doubt be much more favorable.

One comprehensive study published in the *Journal of Biosocial Science* (January 1982) compared women over 35 with women aged 20 to 34 in Hungary (a developed nation) and Mexico and Egypt (relatively undeveloped). It concluded that maternal age does affect a pregnancy, but that the risk is relatively insignificant if a woman is unhampered by low socioeconomic status and poor or relatively absent prenatal care. Finnish researchers reporting in the *International Journal of Gynaecology and Obstetrics* (Volume 19, 1981) found no threat to the health of mothers studied over 40 and only negligibly increased infant risk, given good obstetric care. An examination of nurse-midwife deliveries at New York's Roosevelt Hospital from 1977 to 1981 was described in the *Journal of Nurse-Midwifery* (January/February 1983); when women with preexisting medical conditions were screened out, mothers over 35 were able to deliver successfully and not much differently from younger mothers. This helps explain why midwives are enthusiastic about the over-35 women they see, as are prepared-childbirth instructors.

Iris Kern of the University of the District of Columbia reported in 1983 the results of a study of 75 over-35 mothers. The women were well-educated professionals and experienced few problems with labor and delivery; only 12% had a cesarean section, and all but one child (born with Down's syndrome) were normal and healthy.

Perinatal, or close to birth, deaths seem higher in number for babies of older mothers, but most of these deaths occur in the womb. Once born, the infant of a woman over 35 has as much chance of survival as the infants of younger women. This was the conclusion of a still widely quoted study by Dr. Sidney Kane published in *Obstetrics and Gynecology* in March 1967, and it was confirmed by a South Carolina study published in the same journal 10 years later, in March 1977. The 1982 developed/ developing nations study found a significant increase in perinatal mortality among older mothers in Mexico and Egypt, a greater proportion of whom were socioeconomically at risk; the better-off Hungarian mothers experienced only a marginal rise in perinatal deaths. And the 1981 Finnish report found no increase in perinatal deaths for the over-40 women studied.

In assessing risk, you don't want to lose sight of the absolute figures. The infant mortality rate for all U.S. women as of 1982 was 11 per 1,000 live births—about 1%. Chromosomal defects occur in less than 1% of fetuses. Miscarriage is more common; it happens to between 10% and 15% of pregnant women. (That is, women who know they're pregnant—unrecognized pregnancy loss in the very early weeks may be many times higher.) Maternal mortality is hard to express in terms of percentages—in 1982 it was only 9 per 100,000 live births, less than 1 in 10,000—.01%. If you are at somewhat increased risk in these categories, it still doesn't amount to a very great one. And the figures include all women, even those who, the studies show, contribute most heavily to unfavorable pregnancy outcomes, members of low socioeconomic groups with inadequate care and nutrition.

To assure yourself of the smallest possibility of an age-related complication of pregnancy, follow the simple plan emphasized repeatedly throughout this book. Initiate and maintain good prenatal care and screen for medical disorders and abnormalities of the pregnancy. Then follow the recommendations in the following chapter to keep you and your developing baby healthy, fit, and well-nourished.

CHAPTER 7

FITNESS, NUTRITION, AND DRUGS

Pregnancy doesn't just happen to you. It's something you can actively participate in. The more involved you are, the more comfortable and trouble-free your pregnancy will be and the healthier your baby will be, before and after birth. You might take what you eat and drink and your physical activity for granted when you're not pregnant, but you have to pay attention to these things now that you are.

Fitness

Fitness is a national craze. With everyone on the bandwagon, it's no surprise that fitness in pregnancy is getting a lot of attention now, too. The phenomenally successful Jane Fonda Workout has been adapted to expectant mothers; *Jane Fonda's Workout Book for Pregnancy, Birth, and Recovery* is available as a book, audio or video cassette, or series of classes. Publications as diverse as *The Runner* and *Journal of the American Medical Association* report the benefits of jogging during pregnancy. Actresses and television newscasters, the most highly visible of today's over-35 mothers, extol the benefits of the exercise programs that kept them fit for nine months and made them svelte in record time after delivery.

Keeping fit when you're pregnant goes beyond trendiness. Pregnancy places terrific physical demands on you, and if your labor is typical, you'll find it by far the most strenuous event you ever have or ever will participate in. There's no way to avoid the physical strains of pregnancy. You can, however, prepare for and cope with them better if you condition your body and keep it conditioned throughout your pregnancy.

This is particularly true when you're over 35. You're used to an active, healthy lifestyle. However, your body is less flexible now than it was when you were younger, so you may find it harder to adapt to the physical strains of pregnancy. Your uterine muscles may have lost some of the tone required for efficient labor. And let's face it—staying in shape and controlling weight takes more effort after you hit your mid 30's, pregnant or not. Just like those over-35 actresses and newscasters, you'll have to work harder than most younger women to get back into shape after delivery. If you're physically fit during the pregnancy—or, ideally, before you conceive—these age-related problems will be minimized. It's like a friend of mine who was up, around, and out of the hospital far ahead of schedule after heart bypass surgery at the age of 40. "Sure, it was tough," he said, "but imagine how much worse it would have been if I hadn't been in good shape!"

Exercising while pregnant calls for some caution, however, because of certain changes in your body. Your expanding uterus and its contents place a tremendous strain on your muscles, joints, and ligaments. Your skyrocketing hormone levels have softened your ligaments and loosened your joints. Your center of gravity has shifted and continued to do so. This all makes you more susceptible to injury while exercising. Also, exercise restricts blood flow, and therefore oxygen and nutrients, to the fetus. If your circulation is already impaired by hypertension, pre-eclampsia, or a heart condition, exercise other than the most moderate during pregnancy is not recommended. Kidney disease and diabetes are also contraindications for unnecessary exertion. Exercise can stimulate uterine activity, a special hazard if you're at risk for preterm delivery.

Because of these potential problems, you must clear all exercises and sports activities with your practitioner. This is not the time to begin a new sport or vigorous activity, but you should be able to continue any regimen you're already active in. If you've been really sedentary up until now, you do need to start some moderate exercise. A program of stretching and strengthening routines plus long walks will counteract age-related weakening of muscle tone. Certain types of exercises can place undue strain on already stressed muscles, ligaments, and joints, so don't do any self-designed exercises or any that aren't specifically tailored to pregnant women.

Exercising alone can be boring and hard to stick with on your own. Celia, pregnant at 37, counteracted this syndrome by joining a prenatal exercise program at her local YMCA. Although she'd never been a successful exerciser before, Celia loved the opportunity to be with other big-bellied women, laughing at their common difficulties and sharing pride in their calisthenic abilities. After delivery, Celia found herself hooked on exercise and went back to the Y for a post-partum class for mothers and infants, which not only entertained her but also offered her the company of a peer group, and gave her an opportunity to get herself and her infant out of the house.

Where can you find exercise classes? Like Celia, you can call your local YMCA or YWCA. Alternatively, your prepared-childbirth class will include an exercise program or direct you to one. The hospital or birth center where you plan to deliver is another source, as are private exercise salons. If you think you'd be a successful at-home exerciser, there are many good books on the market outlining pregnancy exercise routines— for instance, the Jane Fonda book already mentioned; *Essential Exercises for the Childbearing Year* by Elizabeth Noble; *You & Me, Baby,* by Susan L. Regnier, based on the YMCA program; and others. The photos in these books of very pregnant exercising women in leotards and tights are definitely reinforcing.

Use good judgment in your fitness activities. As with all exercise, the most important guideline is: don't strain. Do only as much as you find comfortable. If you experience any problems, stop what you're doing and report the symptoms; don't start again till you've got a medical okay. Reportable problems include pain (abdominal, back, leg, etc.), breathing difficulties, and unusual discharge. To be certain you're not interrupting your baby's oxygen supply, make sure you can talk and still breathe easily while exercising. When doing stretching exercises, don't bounce or force the stretch. Flat-on-the-back exercises may leave you lightheaded because of the blood pooled in your legs; if so, cut out these routines, or only move to a more upright position very slowly. Pay special attention to warming up—it takes longer when you're pregnant. If your activity is vigorous enough to burn off calories needed for fetal development, replace them. Don't exercise till you're tired out; that will just add to the problem of pregnancy fatigue. Be consistent. One 60-minute session a week isn't going to help and may harm; aim for 10 to 20 minutes daily. Let common sense be your guideline. Relaxation techniques or exercises can be combined with your fitness routine to round out your sense of well-being.

Your tolerance for exercise will vary from trimester to trimester. You may want to skip very active exercise in the first trimester when you're battling fatigue (some doctors advise against exercise then anyway), and your size will force a slowing down during the final trimester. You may have trouble with weight-dependent exercises, those such as jogging or tennis in which you have to support your body weight. This was the case with Esther, who found running extremely uncomfortable in her second trimester. She switched to swimming, a weight-independent exercise that she was able to continue through the rest of her pregnancy. Stationary bicycling would have been another option. Not all joggers are forced to quit, though. "Pregnant Jogger: What a Record!" headlined the *Journal of the American Medical Association* in July 1981. A 36-year-old mother of six ran four miles per day throughout her seventh pregnancy, slowing down to a four-mile walk the day of delivery after labor began.

You should probably avoid sports that can involve a jarring fall, like skiing or bicycle riding. The reason is not that you might jar the baby loose; women have tried for eons to get rid of unwanted pregnancies this way, and mostly failed. The baby is well cushioned in its amniotic sac. The real danger is your increased vulnerability to injury—of the spine, of joints, of muscles, tendons, and ligaments. And do you really want to cope with pregnancy plus a cast on your leg or arm?

If your partner, friends, or relatives express concern about the effect of your activities on your baby, tell them about an examination of deliveries at Yale-New Haven Hospital in 1977, reported in the *Journal of Reproductive Medicine* (September 1983). Researchers there determined that women who had been active in sports or physical fitness programs had fewer preterm deliveries than inactive mothers. Furthermore, studies of pregnant athletes show that these women usually have shorter labors, fewer problems in pregnancies, and better fetal outcomes unless they maintain highly competitive activity, in which case their pregnancies are more complicated. And their performance actually improves after having babies, according to the journal *The Female Patient* (February 1979).

Years ago, women weren't expected to exercise during pregnancy. Women, in general, weren't active in sports, and not much was known about the benefits of regular exercise. Today it's unusual not to be urged by your practitioner and childbirth instructor to keep yourself fit, especially because of your age. Some Olympic athletes have been pregnant when they won their medals, including June Irwin, who won a bronze medal for platform diving, and Andrea Mead Lawrence, who garnered two gold medals in alpine skiing. Jockey Mary Bacon rode three consecutive races hours before delivering her baby girl. While you're not likely to be competing in the Olympics or the Kentucky Derby during your pregnancy, you can at least keep fit and treat yourself to a much more comfortable pregnancy and a greatly increased ability to labor and deliver efficiently.

Nutrition

Good nutrition during pregnancy is critical to the growth and development of your baby. Vast changes take place as a one-celled ovum rapidly divides and redivides to become, nine months later, an eight-pound baby with billions of cells. A steady supply of nutrients in the necessary amounts is required to fuel this change. Specific systems need specific minerals or vitamins in order to develop properly. And your baby needs to achieve an optimum weight before birth.

No problem, you say? You're fairly well-off and have an adequate diet; malnourishment is exclusively a condition of the poor, the disadvantaged. And the baby will take whatever it needs from you anyway—if not from what you're eating, then from your stored reserves. Wrong on both counts. It's not at all unusual for middle- and upper-class U.S. women to suffer from poor nutrition. In 1975, HEW found one out of three pregnant women to be malnourished. For women not in low socioeconomic groups, the culprit is fad diets, lack of information, or poor habits. A career woman also caring for a home and family has a tendency to skip meals or eat pickup, fast-food style. As for the baby cannibalizing you to meet its needs, it's more like a competition. Your body takes what it needs, too, and may prevail over the baby. Either way, neither of you gets enough.

Inadequate nutrition can have serious consequences for your baby, increasing the risks of being born dead, prematurely, defective, unhealthy, or underweight. Low birth weight is a real threat, making the child more susceptible to infection, developmental problems, and mental retardation or learning disabilities.

Being well nourished is important to you, too. You'll substantially lower your chances of developing complications like infection, hypertension, or anemia. You'll do better in labor and delivery, with less risk of a cesarean. You'll be able to handle the stresses of pregnancy and the postpartum period more successfully. You'll be more capable of breastfeeding. And there is a lot of evidence that well-nourished women are unlikely to develop toxemia, a very serious complication of pregnancy. Since some of these problems occur frequently in over-35 women, good nutrition can be extra insurance for you to avoid difficulties.

Practitioners vary a lot in the amount of nutritional counseling they'll offer. However, there's an increasing awareness of the importance of diet on maternal and fetal health, so you're likely to be given some good guidelines, written and oral. Consultation with a nutritionist may be part of your prenatal routine. If not, and if you want more information, you can seek out a nutritionist yourself. Prenatal classes usually include dietary guidance. There are also a number of published dietary recommendations for pregnant women. Educate yourself about food. Read labels, and know what foods provide which nutrients.

Your basic concern is to eat quality foods, not empty calories, an adequate amount from each of the basic food groups daily. Do not skip meals. You should take in around 2500 calories each day, somewhat less in the first trimester. You need lots of protein (75 to 80 grams a day) to fuel the new cells and tissues being created, especially in the last four months or so of pregnancy. You also need plenty of carbohydrates. Going or staying on a low carbohydrate diet now can prove detrimental to the baby's developing brain and nervous system.

Iron demands are very high, to support the expanding blood volume, to build up the baby's reserves, and to maintain your energy level. You're not likely to be able to meet these needs through diet, so your practitioner will probably prescribe a supplement. Calcium demands, too, are greatly increased. You'll have to take in a quart of milk or its equivalent daily; otherwise, the baby will steal calcium from your bones. It's only myth that you lose calcium from your teeth during pregnancy. A lot of fiber will go a long way toward avoiding or relieving pregnancy-induced constipation and hemorrhoids.

Keep your diet low in fats, and be sure you've got a good daily intake of vitamins and minerals. You especially want a higher intake of B vitamins, folic acid in particular, and you may have started your pregnancy somewhat deficient in them, as many American women do. Your practitioner may prescribe a multivitamin, although that doesn't mean you can forget about a balanced diet. You should *not* take large doses of vitamins during your pregnancy. They can build up in your baby and have negative effects. If you're a vegetarian, you'll have to evaluate your diet very carefully to be sure you're meeting your protein, iron, and vitamin B_{12} needs.

A chart that follows shows how considerable the increased protein, vitamin, and mineral requirements for pregnant and breastfeeding women are.

There's some controversy in obstetric circles about what constitutes acceptable pregnancy weight gain. Until about 10 or 15 years ago, obstetricians routinely advised their patients to gain no more than 20 pounds. The weigh-in was a dreaded feature of each prenatal visit. If a woman gained too much (and many did), at too rapid a rate, she would be put on a low-calorie, low-salt diet, and perhaps given diuretics. It was believed that this would prevent toxemia, linked at the time to extra weight gain. Weight control was also supposed to guarantee an easier delivery and have no ill effects on the baby, who was presumed to make up what was needed from the mother's body. Finally, birth weight wasn't linked to maternal weight gain.

Today, maternal weight gain is considered important to the baby's and the mother's health. Most practitioners believe 24 to 28 pounds is a good average increase and aren't unduly concerned about gains of 30 or 35 pounds. They no longer recommend diuretics and recognize the need for adequate amounts of salt. In cases where dietary control is necessary, calories are

not reduced; instead, high-calorie, low-nutrient foods are eliminated. Toxemia is no longer feared as a side effect of "excessive"
(over 20 pounds) weight gain, salty foods, or water retention.
According to Dr. Tom Brewer, a nationally known and contro-
versial expert on pregnancy and nutrition, inadequate weight
gain and salt intake may actually increase susceptibility to toxemia.

Recommended Daily Dietary Allowances for Women (1980 Revision)

	Age/condition		
	23–50 years	Pregnant	Lactating
Protein (g)	44	+30	+20
Fat-Soluble Vitamins			
Vitamin A (mcg)	800	+200	+400
Vitamin D (mcg)	5	+5	+5
Vitamin E (mg)	8	+2	+3
Water-Soluble Vitamins			
Vitamin C (mg)	60	+20	+40
Thiamine (mg)	1.0	+0.4	+0.3
Riboflavin (mg)	1.2	+0.3	+0.5
Niacin (mg)	13	+2	+5
Vitamin B_4 (mg)	2	+0.6	+0.5
Folacin (mcg)	400	+400	+400
Vitamin B_{12} (mcg)	3	+1	+1
Minerals			
Calcium (mg)	800	+400	+400
Phosphorus (mg)	800	+400	+400
Magnesium (mg)	300	+150	+150
Iron (mg)	18	*	*
Zinc (mg)	15	+5	+10
Iodine (mcg)	150	+25	+50

[Source: Food and Nutrition Board of the National Academy of Sciences/
National Research Council, from *FDA Consumer*, March 1984.]

g = grams
mcg = micrograms
mg = milligrams

* 30–60 mg. of supplemental iron is recommended

Your weight gain during pregnancy should be gradual—
slow, but steady. You should gain slowly for about the first 16 to
20 weeks, and put on about a pound a week after that. If you
were overweight to begin with, or if you gain a lot in early
pregnancy, don't try to reverse this by dieting in the later

trimesters. Remember that your baby has an enormous growth spurt in the last trimester, doubling in size. She or he needs an uninterrupted flow of nutrients at all times so development isn't interfered with at any stage. Worry about losing weight *after* the baby's born. Do not diet while breastfeeding.

You may be especially interested in avoiding extra weight gain during pregnancy because of your age—it'll be that much harder to take it off after birth. Keep in mind that your metabolism declines slightly with age, so you may need fewer calories than younger women to maintain a reasonable weight increase. However, you need just as high an intake of minerals, vitamins, and protein, so you will have to adjust your diet very carefully if you're to eliminate calories safely. It might be just as well not to worry about a reasonable weight gain and plan instead on a good pre- and postpartum exercise regimen to manage the return to your prepregnant poundage and shape.

There were wide variations in weight gain among the women I spoke with. Elaine, 39, added only 20 pounds without making any effort to restrict her increase, as did Anne, 38. Valerie, on the other hand, 35 and 38 when she had her two children, gained 63 and 70 pounds; her obstetrician was not overly concerned because Valerie was well nourished. No practitioner, however, would recommend such a large increase as a matter of course.

By the end of nine months, the weight you've gained is baby-related to approximately this degree:

Full term baby—6 to 8 pounds
Placenta—1 to 1½ pounds
Amniotic fluid—1 to 2 pounds
Enlargement of the breasts—2 to 3 pounds
Uterine enlargement—2 to 3 pounds
Blood volume—4 to 5 pounds

The rest of the weight gain is in the form of stored reserves in your body.

Remember to report any sudden, excessive weight gain—for example, 2 to 5 pounds in the space of a week—to your practitioner. And remember, too, if you're carrying more than one child, your weight gain and calorie/nutrient needs will be correspondingly increased. Finally, reflect on the fact that the good nutrition you establish now could get to be a habit and have lifelong, life-prolonging benefits for you.

Drugs

Just as it's essential to consume foods that will supply your baby with all the required nutrients, it's also essential to stay away from substances that could prove harmful. Almost everything you take in can pass through the placenta to the fetus— not just what you eat, but also what you breathe, what you drink, and what you absorb through your skin. Not everything damages the fetus, but many things might.

Agents that cause malformation when taken in during pregnancy are called teratogens, from the Greek *teras*, "monster." Teratology describes the study of abnormal development as well as congenital malformations. It's hard to gauge the effect of a particular suspected teratogen. It may affect only a very small number of fetuses exposed to it, so it's hard to pinpoint that substance as a cause. Or the mother may have exposed her child to several potential toxins. Which is the guilty one? Sometimes effects take such a long time to show up, no one can remember what was taken when. This happened in the 1970's when many mothers of grown children had to remember if they'd taken the hormone DES when they were pregnant in the 1940's or 1950's. And if the substance triggers a miscarriage, it may not be easy to establish cause, since as many as 15% of recognized pregnancies spontaneously abort in any case.

Only 3% of babies are born with serious abnormalities; only about 3% of these malformations are known to be caused by environmental hazards and drugs. However, the origin of two thirds of developmental defects remains unknown. The fetus is particularly vulnerable during the first three months of its development. First all its cells divide and redivide rapidly; then they begin to specialize, and organs, limbs, and facial features are formed. By the 12th postmenstrual week most structural formations and major organ systems are completed. From then on, they simply grow. If the cells are interfered with or altered during the period of formation, gross abnormalities can result. Unfortunately, this is often a time a woman does not yet know she's pregnant. The fetus may have been developing for four or five weeks before the mother becomes aware of its existence, and those weeks, ironically, are potentially the most stressful for the fetus. But the fetus is not immune to influences in the second and third trimesters, although exposure mostly affects growth, development, and future health ʀ than triggering malformations. The same substance can have different effects at different stages of fetal development, and these effects range in seriousness—from slight, such as permanently yellowed teeth, to extreme, such as mental retardation.

When you're considering exposure to toxins, don't ignore your partner. Men, too, are affected. Sperm production may be altered, thus interfering with fertilization or triggering birth defects. Your chances of miscarriage or stillbirth can be affected by your partner's contact with certain substances. This is a situation you must pay attention to *before* you conceive.

Smoking

Smoking is hazardous to your baby. Are you familiar with the Surgeon General's warning on cigarette packs? The House of Representatives passed a bill in September 1984 calling for four new, rotating warnings. The one relating to pregnancy reads, "Smoking by pregnant women may result in fetal injury, premature birth, and low birth weight." The bill was supported even by the tobacco industry.

A mother who smokes is twice as likely to have a low-birth-weight baby, which we've seen can threaten a baby's survival, future health, and development. Even smokers' babies within the normal weight range weigh less than nonsmokers' babies. It may not seem like much, but a difference of six or eight ounces can be critical to a child born with other difficulties. This is especially important when you consider that smoking also increases the chance of a premature birth. Stillbirth, miscarriage, perinatal death, and placental abnormalities are more likely, too; at least one researcher has reported that smokers are twice as likely as nonsmokers to miscarry (*Obstetrics and Gynecology*, April 1980). These risks go up if you drink as well as smoke. It's not yet clear whether smoking causes congenital defects.

Cigarette smoking affects your baby in two major ways. First, nicotine constricts maternal blood vessels, reducing the amount of oxygen and food passing to the fetus. Each time you smoke a cigarette, for as long as you smoke it, your blood vessels are constricted and your baby is deprived of nourishment. And since nicotine enters your baby's blood vessels, they may become constricted, too. Second, the carbon monoxide in cigarette smoke is absorbed by the blood, in place of the oxygen needed by your baby to build tissues. The effect is twofold: maternal blood vessels pass more carbon monoxide (CO) and less oxygen along through the placenta; fetal blood then captures the CO and keeps it in circulation longer, interfering with absorption of the already reduced oxygen supply. It's a kind of double whammy: nicotine reduces blood flow, therefore oxygen, and carbon monoxide reduces the blood's ability to carry oxygen. If you're hitting your baby with the nicotine/CO combination 10, 20, or 30 times a day, you can see how it will measurably retard your baby's growth.

Nicotine also speeds up your baby's heart rate while you're smoking. And cigarettes depress the breathing activities of an unborn child, so your infant is more likely to have respiratory problems after birth. Some studies have even found physical and mental development problems in older children whose mothers smoked during the last half of pregnancy. If you continue to smoke after your baby's birth, your child will be more susceptible to a variety of illnesses.

How much you smoke and when does make a difference. The babies of lighter smokers are less growth-retarded than those of heavier smokers. Also, if you stop smoking before the fifth month, your baby's development may not be adversely affected at all. Stopping at any time will probably have some beneficial effect, and cutting down to less than 10 a day will certainly help. Note, though, that low tar and nicotine cigarettes do not have lowered levels of carbon monoxide. If you live with a smoker or work in a smoke-filled environment, you need to make an effort to eliminate or reduce that smoke, too.

If you smoke, use your pregnancy to try to break the addiction. Convince yourself that the hazards to your baby are real, then decide to quit. Choose a method that works well for you; go cold turkey, cut down gradually, or join a smoke-ending group. If you're worried about gaining weight when you stop smoking, remember that you're supposed to be gaining now. In fact, the appetite depression that accompanies smoking may interfere with nutrition and adequate weight gain. You can eat more now; just follow the dietary recommendations given earlier. Caffeine and alcohol are often paired with smoking, so restricting their use will help you cut back on cigarettes too. Exercise more and be active.

Cutting out cigarettes will not only benefit your baby but may also free you for life of an expensive and hazardous habit. Of course, you don't want your levels of stress and tension to be so elevated by trying to quit that they pose a threat to your child. Even if you don't eliminate smoking entirely, working toward that goal should cut down your cigarette use substantially.

Alcohol

The dangers of alcohol to a pregnant woman are not as clear-cut as the hazards of smoking. Alcohol does present a teratogenic risk to the developing fetus because it passes through the placenta and enters the baby in the same concentration as it enters in you. Imagine giving your six-month-old a glass of wine or a shot of scotch! That's what you're doing to your unborn child each time you have a drink. Alcohol is processed by the liver, and the immature liver of your baby can't efficiently burn up the alcohol. It circulates through your baby's developing tissues until it is processed.

One constellation of abnormalities—fetal alcohol syndrome—is known to result from the mother's heavy use of alcohol. This condition is found in 30% to 50% of babies born to chronic alcoholic mothers. It results in a pattern of malformations including abnormalities of the eyes, joints, and heart, retarded growth, lowered intelligence, and impaired motor development. Newborns suffer from withdrawal symptoms.

Fetal alcohol syndrome is a risk if the mother drinks as much as 3 to 5 ounces of pure alcohol a day, or 6 to 10 cocktails. (One ounce of pure alcohol equals about 2 ounces of liquor, two 5-ounce glasses of wine, or two 12-ounce bottles of beer.) More moderate use of alcohol, about 2 ounces (four drinks) or more daily seems also to produce mild FAS symptoms in 10% to 20% of infants.

Professionals disagree about the effect of light or occasional drinking; there is some evidence of lower birth weight and a higher miscarriage rate, but nothing has been proven. Again, the risks may be higher if you smoke and drink. One reason it's hard to judge the effects of alcohol is that some women and some fetuses metabolize it differently than others. It is known that alcohol can deplete your body of some vitamins and minerals, a particularly undesirable effect when you're pregnant.

Since alcohol in large doses is known to be harmful to the fetus and can cause problems in moderate doses, it seems sensible to avoid regular use of it during pregnancy. An occasional, nondaily drink before dinner or a glass of wine with it probably presents little risk. Women have been doing it for years before the questions were raised. Never, however, binge drink while pregnant, and forego even that occasional glass of wine when labor is just beginning. It can slow down your uterine contractions and prolong labor.

Caffeine

Lately a lot of controversy has emerged about caffeine. This chemical is found in coffee, tea, sodas, chocolate, some baked goods, and many cold medications. Like alcohol, it passes into the fetal bloodstream in unchanged concentration from your bloodstream. Its hazards are not well established. Very heavy coffee intake (eight cups a day) does increase the risk of spontaneous abortion, stillbirth, and prematurity. Excessive caffeine intake has also been associated with infertility. On the other hand, moderate caffeine consumption has not been documented as having an adverse effect. While an extremely heavy caffeine diet has produced birth defects in laboratory animals, it's not clear if human beings would react the same way. Researchers reporting in 1983 found no correlation between coffee consumption by pregnant women and the birth of malformed babies. The study, published in the *American Journal of Public Health* (December 1983), was conducted in Finland, which has the world's highest per capita coffee consumption. Caffeine does encourage stomach acid, not good if you're bothered by heartburn or indigestion. It also stimulates you to urinate more often, adding to frequent-trips-to-the-bathroom annoyance.

Many drinks such as coffee, tea, and colas can be purchased in caffeine-free form, affording substitutes for the heavy caffeine user. Check all ingredients first for naturally occurring toxins; read your food labels and avoid chocolate. As for cold medications, see the following.

Prescription, Over-the-Counter, and Street Drugs

A study conducted recently by the National Institutes of Health indicated that women take an average of four drugs during pregnancy, excluding nutritional substances such as vitamins. Almost half of the drug use occurred in the first trimester when the potential for damage to the growing fetus is greatest. Most drugs were self-prescribed and presumably sold over the counter. Apparently, these women have not gotten the message: absolutely no drug is safe if you are or might be pregnant, without the sanction of a medical practitioner. This includes substances you might think are so common as to be harmless, such as aspirin, which is considered dangerous in the third trimester because of its association with maternal and infant hermorrhage, impaired fetal circulation, and prolonged gestation and labor. It also includes medications you're already on, like the Pill.

Drugs that are safe and beneficial for you may harm your developing child because they pass over to the fetus and affect it in a different way than how they affect you. The dosage you take is related to your body weight. There's a lot of body to absorb and disperse the drug. Relative to you, your baby is tiny but is receiving the same dosage. Also, your liver breaks down the drug and converts it into usable substances. Your baby can't do this, so the drug stays in the baby's system in its original form and can produce quite a different effect in the infant than in you.

Not all medications are harmful to a developing fetus. Many women have taken drugs during pregnancy and not given birth to a defective child. However, the information on many drugs is incomplete, inconclusive, or completely absent, which is why they're best avoided whenever possible.

The thalidomide tragedy alerted doctors, the public, and drug companies to both the grave threat drugs pose to the unborn child and the difficulty of establishing that threat through testing. Thalidomide was a widely used tranquilizer that at first could be purchased without prescription in Europe. It had passed laboratory tests on pregnant animals. Yet in 1962 it was revealed to be the cause of gross abnormalities in infants' limbs. The drug only has this effect during the period in early pregnancy of about two weeks when the fetal limbs are beginning to develop. The thalidomide discovery has greatly reduced the prescription or recommendation of drugs for pregnant women.

Nevertheless, problems continue to occur. Since June 1983 there has been no FDA-approved drug available in the United States for morning sickness. At that time, Merrell Dow Pharmaceuticals ceased production of Bendectin, a widely prescribed medication for early-pregnancy nausea. Thirteen days earlier, a family had been awarded $750,000 for the birth of a daughter with serious limb deformities; the mother had taken Bendectin during pregnancy. Faced with hundreds of other lawsuits claiming Bendectin-induced birth defects, Merrell Dow chose to halt production of the drug.

Sometimes, however, you need medication—for instance, to control an infection or a chronic disease. Many infections pose serious threats to a developing baby and must be treated. The seriousness of the problem being treated must be weighed against the potential risk to the fetus. Ask your practitioner about the potential effects; the FDA requires that these be listed for prescription medications. If one drug is contraindicated during pregnancy, there may be a safer substitute. In general, though, no drug will be prescribed to a pregnant woman unless there is a clear indication that her life or her health is in jeopardy.

If you took a drug before you knew you were pregnant, you can find out what effect it might have had through your practitioner. He or she will have access to whatever is known about the possible teratogenic effect of a given medication, from the drug company manufacturing it, from major medical centers employing experts in perinatology (the study of fetal development), or from genetic counseling centers. There are very few drugs you might take that are so teratogenic that the medical community would advise an abortion.

Because both infections and drugs can harm a fetus, it's obviously best to work at keeping yourself optimally healthy before you conceive and during your pregnancy so you can avoid both illness and medications.

Illegal drugs—marijuana, cocaine, heroin, speed, and the like—should simply be left untouched during pregnancy. Not much is known about their roles in fetal development, but since other drugs are known to be harmful it's reasonable to assume these are likely to be, too. Why take a chance on something unstudied? Moderate marijuana use has not been shown to harm a fetus, but it hasn't been shown to be safe, either. And you can't be sure you're not getting herbicide- or pesticide-contaminated weed or a few extra unknown substances along with it.

Environmental and Other Hazards

In addition to what you eat and drink and the drugs you may ingest, you must avoid exposure to environmental and occupational toxins, radiation, and a few other sources of chemicals. For most people this is no big problem. You're probably not at much risk for exposure anyway. To avoid radiation, don't have X-rays while you're pregnant or when you may be pregnant. They can seriously damage a fetus, especially in the early months. If diagnostic X-rays are suggested to you for any reason while you're pregnant, put them off if possible until after you deliver, and always protect your abdomen with a lead covering if the X-rays are taken. You certainly don't want your abdomen radiated! X-rays, incidentally, are another example of delayed discovery of teratogenic effect. They were used widely for years before researchers linked them to cancer and birth defects.

You should also be able to avoid most environmental toxins, if you know they're present. There's been a lot of publicity in the past few years about hazardous waste sites and abandoned chemical dumps and their possible effects on pregnant women and unborn babies. Agricultural spraying, too, has been questioned. Toxic substances may be present at your place of work. Little is known for sure about many of these toxins, but again it's best to shun them when possible. See the discussion in Chapter 9 on hazards in the workplace. Be aware of what chemicals you use at home, too, such as dry-cleaning solvents, aerosols, cleaners, insecticides, and garden compounds.

As long as you're avoiding other chemicals, it's probably wise to be wary of many food additives. While none currently used has been shown to be harmful to an unborn child, some haven't been tested thoroughly enough. Your diet should emphasize fresh and unprocessed items.

Finally, you may not think to watch your cosmetics, but remember that toxins can be absorbed into your body through your skin. Some cosmetics contain hormones, a real no-no in pregnancy (DES is a hormone, for example). Find a natural substitute. Your radically altered hormone balance can also produce unpleasant allergic reactions to cosmetics you normally use. And there's evidence you should not dye or bleach your hair during pregnancy; these substances are absorbed through your scalp and may also be teratogenic.

Conclusion

By now, you're saying to yourself there's too much to avoid. Why even try? Because your baby needs as protective and benign an environment as possible in order to grow and develop to his or her maximum potential. You wouldn't blow smoke in your baby's face, measure a martini into her bottle, or give him a tranquilizer, so don't do it now in utero. Remember, however, that very few babies are born with serious defects, and the odds that something you do—especially if you're exercising reasonable care—will cause a malformation are very far out in left field. There's a lot of pressure today on expectant mothers; as genetic counselor Elsa Reich expressed it to me, "Pregnancy has become a pathological state." Don't spend your pregnancy in a state of anxiety or guilt about that glass of wine last weekend or the cigarette you smoked Saturday night. Just don't make them a daily habit.

The basic thing to keep in mind when considering fitness, nutrition, and drug use is this: establish habits that are safe and beneficial for pregnancy prior to it, if at all possible. Years of stored-up nutrients are called on to help sustain a fetus. Weight loss, weight control, and dietary limits can prevent or eliminate some age-related risks such as hypertension and complications of pregnancy. This does *not* include fad or crash diets, which weaken muscle tone and can adversely affect your reproductive system. Weight control and fitness can start you off in as good physical shape as your younger sisters when you conceive. A thorough physical before you become pregnant is a good idea to screen out or pinpoint any problems and is recommended strongly for anyone over 35 just starting an exercise routine. Always keep in mind that you might be pregnant without knowing it if you're sexually active and not using birth control, or using it in a haphazard way. Proceed cautiously, as if you have conceived, remembering how vulnerable a fetus is during that first month.

Following these guidelines, you ought to be able to relax and enjoy your pregnancy knowing you're doing what you can to nurture and protect your unborn child.

CHAPTER 8

BIRTH METHODS AND CHOICES

The options in birth methods and attendants made possible by modern technology are dazzling. You and your partner should use all the vast information at hand to make your choice for delivery one you are comfortable with and confident in.

The Development of Modern Obstetrics

Before modern medicine entered the world of pregnancy and childbirth, that realm belonged, nearly exclusively, to women. The laboring wife was attended by other women and, often, by a female midwife. In European societies, men were routinely barred from the scene of labor, except for male doctors, who were admitted, but only when absolutely necessary. Midwives in the Middle Ages even had to swear to an oath administered by the Church, which included an agreement to avoid the presence of men during labor. During this time the "lithotomy" or lying-on-the-back position was unknown. A laboring woman simply assumed the position she felt most comfortable in. The birthing stool was used widely. This was a stool with a rim to support the woman in labor but with no center to allow delivery of the infant.

Louis XIV of France revolutionized the birth process when he engaged a male, Julien Clement, to attend one of his mistresses during her labor. This lady delivered lying down, either because Clement preferred it that way for his own convenience or so that a hidden Louis could better observe the procedure. In any event, men had entered the birth chamber for the first time and women had begun to give birth on their backs.

This innovation might have died out had it not been for the

invention of the obstetrical forceps by the Chamberlen family of doctors in the late 1500's. Forceps, also called "iron hands," had been used in ancient Egyptian and Hindu cultures, but knowledge of them had been lost. The Chamberlens went to great lengths to keep the forceps a family secret. They carried the device ceremonially into the birth chamber in a large carved and gilded box, which was not opened until the laboring woman had been blindfolded. The patient never laid eyes on the instrument used to deliver her child. While the Chamberlen family managed to keep exclusive possession of the forceps for over a century, stories tell us that in the 1700's one of their number betrayed them by selling the information about the instrument to an outsider. Its use became widespread.

Forceps transformed childbearing. Their impact was twofold. First, they hastened the replacement of female midwives by male doctors. Most midwives couldn't afford forceps, and even if they could, only male doctors knew how to use the device, and these doctors wouldn't share their knowledge with female midwives. Second, the use of forceps required the lithotomy, or lying down, position.

These changes were solidified in Western society during the 1800's. Medical schools, established in the United States by the end of the 18th century, admitted only men, and thus women were shut off from professional knowledge of obstetrical advances. With the advent of anesthesia in the 1840's, chloroform and ether became available and their use during labor acceptable after Queen Victoria allowed chloroform to be administered to her during the birth of her child in 1853. Later, nitrous oxide or "laughing gas" was used for laboring women. Other 19th-century medical advances included ergot to induce contractions, the stethoscope to listen to the fetal heartbeat, instruments for dilating the cervix, and silver nitrate for infants' eyes.

As medical techniques developed, obstetrics became more interventionist and in the second half of the 19th century acquired the status of a specialty. By 1900, the upper and middle classes in the United States agreed with the medical profession that childbirth was a condition requiring medical control. The use of drugs, instruments, and even surgery had come to be expected. And women, who were viewed as hysterical,* unsta-

---

* The word *hysteria* comes from the Greek word *hysteron*, or "uterus." Both Greek and Egyptian physicians taught that hysteria—a female disorder—was caused by a uterus roaming around in the body. Once surgery made it possible, hysterectomy was recommended as a cure for hysteria.

ble, and incapable of accurately noting and reporting symptoms (which in any case were likely to be imaginary), could certainly not oversee such a sophisticated process.

In spite of all this, the concept of hospital birth was rejected at the turn of the century. It was expensive, affordable only by the well-to-do or on a charitable basis for the poor. The middle classes stayed home. Hospitals weren't easy to get to, unless you lived in a city, and they were considered unsafe. Disease could be contracted there, and people feared that extra, unnecessary obstetrical precautions were likely to be taken.

Certainly hospitals had *not* been safe until the latter part of the 1800's. Before then, many hospitalized women in maternity wards had died of childbirth, or puerperal, fever. The cause was unknown until the 1840's, when Dr. Oliver Wendell Holmes in the United States and Dr. Ignaz Semmelweis in Vienna, Austria, both concluded that the fever was a contagion spread by doctors themselves. Physicians and medical students, incredibly, came directly from diseased patients and autopsies to the maternity ward and examined their female patients without washing their hands first. Semmelweis noted that women attended by hospital midwives (who had no contact with other hospital patients, dead or alive) or who delivered before reaching the hospital had significantly lower rates of puerperal fever. Incidences of the fever dropped convincingly after Semmelweis ordered medical students to scrub their hands in disinfectant before examining maternity patients. Unfortunately, the theories of Holmes and Semmelweis were not adopted until after the 1860's. When they were, hospital delivery became much safer.

The practice of obstetrics and the process of childbearing continued to change in the 20th century. Early in the 1900's birth and death statistics became available, and it grew apparent that maternal and infant mortality rates were quite high in the United States—higher, in fact, than in many other countries. In 1917 reports revealed that only tuberculosis killed more women aged 15 to 44 than childbirth. Many physicians urged the upgrading of obstetric education and training. Once again, midwives were shut off from much of what little training had been available to them. Doctors stressed the difficulties of obstetrics, the skills needed, the complexity of the specialty.

Further technological advances did make the practice of

obstetrics more complex. Twilight Sleep was introduced early in the 1900's. Heralded as "painless childbirth," it was a light sleep produced by an injection of an amnesiac drug and morphine. Administration of this and other drugs during labor often meant the use of forceps during delivery, which in turn necessitated the episiotomy. Cesarean sections, too, grew common in 1930. Further advances were made in the use of anesthetics and analgesia. Blood transfusions could be given. X-rays could reveal cephalo-pelvic disproportion, a fetal head too large for the mother's pelvis. All of these procedures required the presence of a doctor, who naturally chose to perform them in a hospital.

These medical developments inevitably moved childbirth from the home to the hospital. While hospitals were still shunned in 1908, by 1940 half of all U.S. births took place in a hospital; the proportion was much higher in urban areas. Home births attended by midwives had remained popular among the rural and immigrant female population which, as the 20th century progressed, diminished. Cars were now becoming universally available to transport the laboring woman to a medical center. By the mid 1970's only 1% of all births in the United States were taking place *outside* a hospital.

In spite of all medical advances, however, not much could be done to help a problem pregnancy 30 years ago. Fewer women died due to childbirth, but there was little way to tell if the fetus had a problem during gestation or delivery or to help an infant born with a medical disorder. That has changed, and continues to change, radically. In fact, the fetus is now considered to be a patient as well as the pregnant woman.

In 1900 the maternal death rate in the United States was 1 for every 100 pregnancies. The average woman at that time had 5 pregnancies, so her chances of dying because of a pregnancy were 1 in 20. Today the maternal death rate is less than 1 for every 11,000 pregnancies. A woman who has 2 pregnancies faces a pregnancy-related death risk of only 1 in 5500. Similarly, in 1915 the infant death rate was 1 for every 10 live births. Today that rate is 1 for every 91 live births. Both rates continue to drop each year.

As medical developments occurred, childbirth became more technological and less personal. Inevitably, a reaction set in. First, interest grew in "natural" or prepared childbirth, with an emphasis on drug- and instrument-free labor and delivery.

In the 1940's, an obstetrician named Grantly Dick-Read toured the United States explaining his method of "natural" childbirth. His book *Childbirth Without Fear* was published in 1944. The Dick-Read method involved relaxation routines and psychological conditioning to remove the fear and tension of labor. This wasn't enough however, to revise the standard anesthetized hospital routine.

Meanwhile, a "psychoprophylactic" method was being developed in Russia based on Pavlov's findings of conditioned response. Pregnant women were taught basic breathing techniques to negate the pain of uterine contractions. Fernand Lamaze, a French obstetrician, observed this procedure in 1951 and started using it when he returned to Paris. An American woman named Marjorie Karmel gave birth in Paris in 1955 using the Lamaze technique. She introduced it to the American public in 1959 with the publication of her book *Thank You, Dr. Lamaze*. A year later Karmel, Elisabeth Bing, and Dr. Benjamin Segal founded the organization that spread the word and the teaching of Lamaze birth: ASPO, the American Society for Psychoprophylaxis in Obstetrics. ASPO worked within the existing system, pushing the concept of a mother's being able to participate in the birth of her child without medication and— revolutionary for American obstetrics—having the father remain present throughout the delivery. Resistance by the medical profession was considerable at first. However, over time, the Lamaze method became almost *de rigueur* for middle-class couples, and it was a rare hospital that did not sanction Lamaze deliveries.

Through Lamaze training, husbands and wives became accustomed to regulating certain aspects of labor and delivery, rather than acquiescing to hospital- and doctor-directed birth. This evolved into a demand for even greater control over the birth process. Routine hospital procedures such as enemas, preps, stirrups, and arm restraints were challenged. And then other prepared approaches developed.

Dr. Robert Bradley advocates a method which adds to breathing and relaxation lessons a focus on the entire experience of pregnancy and childrearing and on individual response to the body's messages, as well as a consumer-oriented approach to the hospital. While it is similar to Lamaze, the Bradley method is more open to individual approaches, and yet may emphasize drug-free delivery more intensely; Dr. Bradley states in his book, *Husband-Coached Childbirth*, that teachers of his method lose certification if their rate of unmedicated births drops below 90%.

The method advocated by English childbirth educator Sheila Kitzinger emphasizes touch relaxation, an individual approach, and the psychological and sexual facets of the birth experience. Kitzinger describes this approach in her books, *The Experience of Childbirth* and *Giving Birth*. Other orientations toward childbirth include yoga, hypnotism, acupuncture, and decompression of the abdomen in a kind of enveloping bubble. The latest approach is Michel Odent's labor under water, practiced in a French hospital with a shallow pool of warm, unsterilized, additive-free tap water. Immersion is said to facilitate the first stage of labor. Most women leave the pool during delivery, but some babies have actually been born under water, reportedly with no ill effects.

Concern for the baby's birth experience grew after the 1975 U.S. publication of Dr. Frederick Leboyer's book *Birth Without Violence*. The Leboyer approach advocates gentle handling of the newborn infant in order to reduce birth trauma. The method includes the use of dim light, whispered voices, placement of the just-born baby on its mother's abdomen, gentle massage, and a warm bath. Concern for the newborn's emotional well-being has fostered an emphasis on bonding—establishing an emotional connection immediately after birth between the infant and each of its parents.

In a radical shift from obstetrics as practiced in the 1950's, the emphasis has now turned to "family-centered childbirth." Fathers and siblings are included as important participants; bonding with the infant is facilitated; delivery is designed, when possible, to be non-technological and in a comfortable setting. Family-centered birth can take place in a hospital or in an independent birthing center. The natural extension of this is to have the ultimate family-centered birth: at home. A still small home-birth movement has been growing over the past 10 years or so. Proponents view it as the definitive way to avoid unwanted intervention in the birth process, and it represents a return full circle to those days when few women delivered outside the home. Let's take a closer look at today's childbirth scene.

Preparing for Birth

It is a rare mother these days who hasn't undergone some form of childbirth preparation. This does not mean that virtually every woman embraces "natural" childbirth. It does mean that most women educate themselves to some degree about the process of labor and delivery. This is only sensible. In our society we almost never come to our first pregnancy having observed another woman in labor; we have no first-hand knowledge about what's likely to happen. And before you became pregnant yourself, you probably found other women's tales of pregnancy, labor, and delivery to be so extraordinarily boring you scarcely listened to them at all. Any "real" experience of labor is usually what has been gleaned from Hollywood and TV, which feature the sudden onset of severe labor, often in response to a traumatic event, followed by agonized moans and screams listened to but not observed by the waiting father for a wrenchingly long time. Talk about negative conditioning!

This highly unrealistic portrait of labor fosters our ignorance. Unfortunately, though, ignorance will not produce a blissful labor—quite the opposite. As Dick-Read observed, ignorance produces fear, which creates tension, increasing perception of pain. If you tense up during each contraction, you counteract the work the uterus is doing to dilate the cervix, thereby lengthening your labor. This is particularly undesirable when you're at risk for a somewhat longer labor anyway because of your age. Preparation for childbirth is based on the premise that knowledge of what to expect will reduce fear and the resultant tension.

At childbirth classes, you'll meet other expectant couples and have a chance to share physical and emotional feelings with them. When you spend all day out in the world with "normal," nonpregnant people, you can feel more comfortable in a room full of women the same strange shape as you. Your partner, too, can be reassured to find he's not the only man around living with a woman in this condition. This can be especially important if none of your friends is pregnant or has been anytime recently.

Your childbirth class will also outline what to expect at your local hospital. Some classes include a tour of the hospital maternity center. If yours doesn't, call the hospital and arrange for a tour on your own. Most hospitals have regularly scheduled tours for expectant parents. Be sure to do this well in advance of your due date, in case of early labor.

Birth classes vary a lot in how much they inform you about labor medications and complications. Some approaches emphasize the natural, normal process of labor and delivery and the avoidance of anesthetics and analgesics. This is especially true of the Lamaze and Bradley methods. Critics say that these result in guilt-ridden women who have had a perfectly successful delivery but feel they've failed if they've asked for or accepted a painkiller of any kind. Kate, for instance, accepted a shot of Demerol during transition because she was no longer able to relax between contractions; she continued to feel each contraction and pushed effectively throughout delivery, but felt guilty each time her husband John described the birth to friends as "natural."

Advocates say that women have been conditioned to accept pain medication that is often unnecessary and bad for the baby, depressing its newborn reactions and its ability to nurse and connect with its environment. Both sides have valid points. The most sensible approach is an honest, practical one.

You're very vulnerable during labor, susceptible to suggestion (either pro or con medication), and mentally handicapped for decision making. Your labor coach should be prepared to help you make a decision when you're in the throes of labor should the question of painkillers arise. You may feel confusion like that of Valerie, who—at 35 and then 38—felt unduly influenced in both her labors. The first time she was pressured to accept medication while her husband/coach was briefly out of the room. He refused it for her when he returned. The second time, during a particularly difficult labor, Valerie was urged to refuse painkillers. This time her husband did accept the medication for her. Both decisions, Valerie later agreed, were the right ones for her, but she was unable to make them at the time.

It also helps to be informed about labor complications. This doesn't raise fears; it dispels them. You and your partner need to know about such things as fetal distress, induction and augmentation of labor, and the use of forceps, episiotomies, and cesarean sections. You should also be sure to discuss them with your pratitioner. Your expectations for labor and delivery can suddenly come unraveled. The medical personnel attending you may be predisposed toward more intervention because of perceived difficulties with older births, especially first-time ones. If you're told during labor that some form of intervention is necessary, you should know when and why that procedure is indicated and what the alternatives are.

Some prepared-childbirth advocates speak, as Dr. Lamaze did, of "painless" childbirth, but I personally know no woman who describes her labor and delivery as painless. Expecting mere "discomfort" in labor can make the actual experience a real shock and threaten the control you need to keep on top of or flow with the contractions.

Hospitals often offer prepared-childbirth courses. However, they may emphasize acceptance of standard hospital procedures plus intervention techniques. If you know or expect you will have a cesarean delivery, you may find special preparation classes and support groups in your community, which will be useful in addressing the special needs of both you and your partner. You may also find special classes and groups if you find yourself experiencing a high-risk pregnancy. Other sources of classes include the YMCA, maternity centers, local community health agencies, the Red Cross, and yoga centers. The La Leche League offers help in preparing for breastfeeding.

Many classes go beyond preparation for labor and delivery. One excellent series of courses offered by Pam Tozier, a childbirth instructor/labor room nurse in my community, includes not only regular or refresher Lamaze but also classes about pregnancy fitness, classes about cesarean section, and a class for siblings and grandparents about the forthcoming baby. There are also classes about postpartum shaping up, infant first aid, and breastfeeding. All aspects of delivery are investigated, such as fetal monitoring and IV's, birthing options, and medications (explained by an anesthesiologist). Movies showing vaginal and cesarean delivery are shown, and descriptions of deliveries by new parents are offered.

A number of women do prepare thoroughly for labor and delivery on the first pregnancy but are quite unmotivated to do so for the second. Most regret this after the fact, feeling that they would have coped better had they been retrained. Anne, for instance, had such a difficult second delivery at age 33 when she failed to refresh her Lamaze techniques or to exercise regularly that she prepared and exercised with dedication for her third delivery at 38, even more than for her first. The final labor and delivery were appreciably easier than the preceding two. There's no reason not to be as well prepared for a subsequent pregnancy as for a first; you may even need it more, depending on the variations in your labor.

Does prepared childbirth actually help? Unquestionably, yes. That was the conclusion reached by a controlled study of Lamaze and unprepared delivering mothers reported in the June 1978 issue of *Obstetrics and Gynecology*. There was not much difference in the amounts of medication used or in the length of labor. While Lamaze mothers pushed more effectively, speeding up the second stage of labor, it was slowed down since forceps were used less often for them. Non-Lamaze mothers had only half as many spontaneous deliveries, four times as many cesareans and three times as many cases of toxemia. For the Lamaze mothers, prematurity was cut by one half, perinatal mortality by one quarter, and fetal distress by one fifth over the control group. Prepared childbirth proved decidedly beneficial.

Choosing Your Birth Setting

You have three basic settings to choose from in deciding where you want to give birth: the hospital, a birthing center—either part of or completely separate from a hospital—or home.

Hospital Birth

This remains the most widely selected birth setting. Your choice of hospital is tied in with your choice of practitioner: you can't give birth in a hospital where your doctor or midwife has no staff association. Most women first choose their practitioner, and from that choice follows the choice of hospital. However, there are advantages to doing it the other way around: surveying hospitals close to you, choosing the one that offers you the birth experience you want, and then choosing a practitioner who can attend you there.

Almost everyone in the childbirth field agrees that hospitals have become sensitive to consumer demand. Medical centers need to fill their beds, so they're much more willing now than in the past to accommodate your requests. This means you should review your hospital's maternity policies and routines, decide what changes you want, and get an agreement providing for them beforehand. Your doctor is key in this: he or she has to go along with any special arrangements you request. Your doctor's specific orders for your case are supposed to prevail, but in their absence, standing hospital procedures may be followed.

The problem with the old, standard hospital delivery was that it made the laboring woman feel isolated, alienated, and dehumanized. A woman was fitted into the prescribed routine instead of the routine being adjusted to best help her through the particular circumstances of her birth. This of course made labor more difficult and increased postpartum maladjustment. There is now much more concern for the individual woman, especially since she is likely to have a pretty good idea of what she wants in labor and since she is likely to have a support person to speak up for her when she may find it hard to do so herself.

Here are some things you may want to ask your hospital and your doctor:

- Can you preregister for admission so you and your partner can proceed without delay to the labor area? Can you walk instead of being placed in a wheelchair?
- Are there any standard prepping procedures—an enema or shaving of the pubic hair?
- Can you eat and drink during labor? Can you suck ice chips?
- Can you move around freely during labor? Assume any position you want?
- Can you arrange for a private labor room? Can you deliver in this room?
- Who can be with you in the labor room? During exams? In delivery? Husband? Children? Other family members? Friends?
- What technology/intervention from the following list is used during labor, and to what extent can you avoid it? (IV, external and internal fetal monitoring, labor-augmenting drugs, artificial rupture of membranes, anesthesia and analgesics, episiotomy, forceps, vacuum extractor.)
- Is the nursing staff trained in the method of childbirth you plan to use? Are they supportive?
- Can you deliver in the position of your choice? Are stirrups and straps used for arms and legs?

- Can your partner be present for a cesarean delivery? Do you have a choice of anesthetics for the procedure?
- What is the routine for newborns? Will you be given your baby immediately? Can you nurse right away? Will the baby be removed to the nursery, or is there rooming-in? Can you nurse on demand?
- Is there rooming-in for the baby's father? If not, can he visit any time? Can siblings visit?
- Is breastfeeding encouraged?
- How soon can you leave the hospital?

Alternative Birthing Centers

If a lot of the answers to the above questions are opposite to what you want for your birth experience, it might be easier to look around for a birthing or maternity center than to try to change a lot of your hospital's procedures. Alternative birthing centers have been developed in response to consumer demand for a homelike birth atmosphere and are designed to attract couples who would otherwise opt for home birth.

There are two types of birth centers: in-hospital and out-of-hospital. Both emphasize birth as a family experience conducted in whatever way the parents want it to be. Rooms are homelike, without all the technological apparatus found in a traditional labor room. You'll spend your entire stay at the center in this room: you labor, deliver, recover, and sleep there, as you would in your own bedroom at home. Also, as it would be at home, you may have whomever you want join you during labor and delivery, including siblings and unrelated friends. You can bring comfortable things from home, like pillows and nightgowns and records or tapes. Labor and birth are very messy, though, so save your favorite bedwear for after delivery. A midwife or nurse will follow your progress closely. While fetal heartbeat will be checked regularly, there will be no electronic fetal monitoring or IV's. You'll be encouraged to walk around during labor, and you can deliver in whatever position feels best for you. You will not be medicated.

After birth, you'll be able to nurse your baby immediately and keep the baby with you throughout your stay. The baby's father can also room in. Siblings and grandparents can visit whenever you like. Your stay will probably be quite short, maybe only 12 hours after delivery, with home-care follow-up. Birth centers usually also provide you with prenatal care counseling and infant-care guidance.

To be eligible for an alternative birthing center, you'll have to experience a normal pregnancy with no indications of complications. You'll be transferred from an alternative birthing center to a regular hospital setting should certain problems arise during pregnancy or delivery, such as high blood pressure, breech presentation, or premature labor. You may also be deemed ineligible for an out-of-hospital birth center if you're over 39 or over 35 and having your first child, no matter how normal and uncomplicated your pregnancy may seem to be. This leaves you with only the in-hospital birthing center as an alternative. If you have a choice of hospitals, check them out first. There can be a tendency at some hospitals to transfer you quickly to the traditional maternity section as soon as your labor seems to be progressing "unsatisfactorily" or taking "too long." You'll be particularly at risk for this approach because of your age. Be sure there's more to the center than homey-looking rooms; make certain that your hospital really is committed to the alternative birth concept and procedure, if that's what you've decided you want.

Home Birth

The new home-birth movement begun in the late 1960's has been growing since then. While the numbers of people opting for home birth may not be too great, they've created a hot controversy in obstetrics. Most doctors and hospitals are vehemently opposed to home birth and also alarmed that increasing numbers of parents are choosing it. One of their reactions has been to provide in-hospital care that simulates home-type birth—the alternative birthing centers discussed above.

Is home birth safe? The data are scanty and contradictory. Unplanned home birth is highly risky. When home-birth statistics include unplanned births, the figures show extremely unfavorable neonatal mortality figures. A study of 1,296 home births in North Carolina reported in the *Journal of the American Medical Association* (December 1980) found 120 neonatal deaths per 1,000 in unplanned, professionally unattended home births, compared with a figure of 6 per 1,000 for planned home deliveries attended by a physician or lay midwife. Hospital births showed a neonatal death rate of 12 per 1,000; when extremely high risk infants weighing less than 2,000 grams were excluded from these figures, the hospital neonatal death rate was 7 per 1,000.

The problem comes with the sudden emergency, when life-saving technology is needed instantly to prevent the baby's death or brain damage. Situations like this do occur without warning, and to women who are healthy, fit, and have had a normal pregnancy and early labor. For those who choose home birth, the psychological experience seems to balance out this risk.

As an over-35 mother, home birth will not be recommended for you, especially if you're over 40 or having your first child. The statistical odds of complications occurring are higher for you than for younger mothers, and your baby is considered premium—perhaps irreplaceable should the rare obstetric disaster occur. If home birth appeals to you, check around for a good in-hospital alternative birthing center; this might offer the best of both worlds.

Choosing Your Birth Team

Most women in the United States are attended by an obstetrician during delivery, although midwifery is being revived. Your choice of practitioner will be influenced by the type of birth and birth setting you want. Of course, you may not have that worked out when you first become pregnant and are seeking to start prenatal care. In that case, you'll probably look for an obstetrician.

Physicians

Your first choice may be your current gynecologist or family practitioner. This is fine if you have a good relationship with her or him and if the two of you have a compatible approach to health care. If you don't already have a doctor, you'll have to choose from among those mentioned by your friends, by other pregnant women or parents, or by someone you know on the staff of a local hospital. Interview a doctor before you decide to stick with him or her for the next nine months. Make sure you can talk with the doctor, ask questions, get cogent answers, and that he or she won't put you off or treat you like an inferior.

Obstetricians used to treat their patients customarily in a father-child, superior–inferior manner. Today this attitude is unacceptable, and most practitioners now welcome informed, participating patients.

You'll also want to be sure your doctor is supportive of over-35 pregnancy. Don't sign up with a doctor who expects you to have a more complicated and difficult labor, simply because of your age. This can mean a more technological birth for you and can make you more anxious and less normal-feeling during pregnancy as well. Younger doctors *may* be less likely to be afflicted with paternalism and age prejudice, although it's not guaranteed.

Once you've found an obstetrician you can communicate with, check to see if your ideas about pregnancy and childbirth mesh well with his or hers. You're not trying to grill the doctor; just get a sense of his or her philosophy and approach. You will need to know what the doctor's hospital affiliation is and who covers for the doctor when she or he is not on call. Labor doesn't happen on schedule, so the backup obstetrician may attend your delivery. "If I had to do it again," said an acquaintance of mine, "I'd make sure my doctor had an associate. My obstetrician was out of town when my baby was born."

Note how many women are in the waiting room. If you must wait a long time for your visit to begin, and if there are too many patients, these may be signals that the practitioner will be too rushed to answer your questions in a helpful, unhurried way.

Midwives

There are two types of midwives in this country: lay and nurse. A lay midwife can assist at home births only. She or he generally has no formal training or professional midwifery education, so there is no uniformity of knowledge or skill among lay midwives. A nurse–midwife is a registered nurse who has completed a one- or two-year midwife-education program and then passed a certification exam. Some nurse–midwives are affiliated with hospitals, staffing clinics and alternative birthing centers. Others work at out-of-hospital maternity centers or conduct private practices backed up by obstetricians. Some even practice with doctors, providing care for normal pregnancies.

Nurse–midwives are oriented toward family-centered birth with an emphasis on birth as a normal physiological process. Nurse–midwives offer their clients (not "patients") emotional support, guidance, encouragement, attention, and time. They can provide all your prenatal care. A nurse–midwife will be with you and your partner throughout labor and will do everything possible to help you both achieve the type of birth experience you want.

Since nurse–midwives have been trained to facilitate normal delivery, they are much less inclined than obstetricians to intervene technologically, especially in the case of longer labors. They are, however, prepared to recognize complications and will have backup medical assistance available. Be sure to ask what those arrangements are, when a doctor will be called in, and who the doctor(s) will be. If you're concerned about the over-managing of labor and delivery, particularly for the over-35 woman, a nurse–midwife might be a good choice for you—if you can find one in your area. There aren't too many of them yet, but their numbers are growing as the word spreads among women of the time, attention, and support nurse–midwives offer.

If you can't afford a private physician or can't find or afford a nurse–midwife, your community probably offers several alternatives. Public health agencies or nurses can provide prenatal care. Hospitals usually run an affiliated low-cost or free maternity clinic. Don't let lack of funds interfere with early and continuing prenatal care.

Putting It All Together

Whatever your choices for pregnancy and childbirth, remember that there are many to be made. Pregnancy, labor, and delivery are intense, personal experiences, for both you and your partner. You can plan that experience, to a great degree, to suit yourselves, although the plan won't always follow the expected scenario as events unfold. Still, if you don't make choices, someone else will, and you might not care for the result. You're the consumers—paying for and using services—so you can decide what you want and ask for it. You're older, wiser, and used to arranging things the way you want them. In today's obstetrical climate, that should be no obstacle.

In making choices, you'll find yourself in the middle of two opposing trends. On the one hand you are confronted with increasingly aggressive medical intervention in the childbirth process; on the other hand you encounter a strong advocacy for a personalized, nontechnological birth experience. What may seem like technological overkill to some may be, for others, the only means to a successful childbirth.

One reason women have become free to opt for late childbearing is because the risks that might attend them can be identified and managed. Like many other mothers who have needed assistance during pregnancy and births, I myself feel nothing but gratitude for the help that brought me and my babies through the rough spots. Whatever the method, a successful outcome is highly likely.

CHAPTER 9

PREGNANCY ON THE JOB

Back in the old days, 20 or 30 years ago, a pregnant woman did not stay on the job (if she had one) much beyond the fifth or sixth month. Pregnancy was not considered appropriate for the workplace. Today the majority of American women work outside the home—out of choice and economic necessity—and see no reason to stop simply because they become pregnant. This is particularly true of the new older mothers. In 1980, 80% of the over-35 women who had a first birth were employed in the year before delivery. Of all the women 30 to 44 who gave birth to any child—first, second, or nineteenth—from June 1982 to June 1983, 40% were employed, 34% of them in professional or managerial positions. You're likely to be one of them.

Does employment outside the home increase your risk of obstetric complications? Would your unborn child benefit if you stayed at home? No, according to a report on the outcomes of over 11,000 pregnancies published in the June 1984 issue of the *Journal of Occupational Medicine*. Researchers compared women who worked throughout pregnancy with housewives who were not employed at any time during pregnancy; babies born to both groups were similar in Apgar scores, birth weight, prematurity, use of the special care nursery, and rates of malformation and perinatal death. The housewives were more likely to have a low weight gain during pregnancy. The conclusion was that working to term does not in itself make pregnancy more risky. In fact, the U.S. Public Health Service reported in 1984 that the age-related risk of an unfavorable pregnancy outcome is actually reduced if an older mother is professionally employed, as most first-time over-30 mothers are.

Integrating pregnancy with your job involves some special considerations. You'll have to inform your employer and make arrangements for the necessary leave. The physical and psychological strains of pregnancy will force some adjustments in the way you handle your job and relationships with co-workers. You'll have to sensitize yourself to occupational hazards that could pose dangers for your unborn child and educate yourself about your legal rights and available maternity benefits. Careful financial planning is called for if your income is going to cease temporarily while the expenses mount.

Adapting to Pregnancy at Work

The first person at the office to tell about your pregnancy is your immediate boss. Do not tell co-workers, even those who are good friends, until after you've notified your superior. Plan this conversation ahead of time. Wait until you're past the first trimester, with its higher chance of miscarriage, and are about to start showing. Explain that you plan to continue working (if you do), and discuss your need for time off to accommodate monthly prenatal visits and diagnostic tests such as amniocentesis. If necessary, state when you expect to begin maternity leave and when you anticipate returning. Don't lock yourself into any plans this soon, though. Many women find that circumstances dictate a change in their original plans. You also need to know what benefits your company offers before you can decide what's feasible.

After you've told your boss, and around the time you begin to show, you can announce your pregnancy to your co-workers. If you're fortunate, your condition will be treated matter-of-factly or with moderate, friendly interest. But you may encounter oversolicitousness, paternalism, or disapproval. Now that pregnant women at work are not unusual, you're more likely to be treated normally. Still, some of your co-workers will relate to you more as a pregnant woman than as a professional colleague. You may find this hard to deal with.

As someone who worked during both pregnancies, I would rather not have had the "pregnant body image" with me in the workplace. I have always been my professional self at work. Into this professional self go such qualities as competence and unemotional decision making, together with a more conservative mode of dress and a more formal way of relating to people. I don't bury my personality at work, but I've always put constraints on it. When people began relating to me differently due to my pregnancy, asking all sorts of personal questions and affecting paternalism, I found it harder to keep my professional self intact.

On the other hand, many of the women I spoke with were quite at ease being pregnant at work. Their employers were supportive and very flexible about leave arrangements. Esther, 39, a manager at a large insurance company, said her co-workers looked on her as a role model; no one acted as though it was inappropriate for her to be pregnant and working. Gail, 37, felt that by continuing to work and remaining active she promoted belief in the competence of pregnant women and the viability of older motherhood. She felt confirmed in her professional identity while simultaneously entering a new stage.

Your attitude and appearance can do a lot to ensure you are treated professionally. Don't act differently; don't discuss symptoms and complaints, even when asked; don't ask for or accept special treatment. Pay special attention to your appearance. Stay well groomed. Invest in some good maternity clothes that are appropriate for the office, and wear them before your regular clothes become unattractively snug.

Pregnancy on the job does require some psychological adjustments, especially during the early months. If you're used to performing a job competently, you may be distressed by feelings of ambivalence and detachment. You have to make a greater effort to perform up to your usual standards. You're not quite sure exactly how you're going to integrate career and family, and you worry about it. If you're experiencing early-pregnancy nausea and fatigue that interfere with your job performance, you may feel guilty and drive yourself to overcompensate. In the middle months of pregnancy, you'll feel more comfortable physically. This is a good time to make childcare arrangements and start planning your leave and postpregnancy work schedule.

The final trimester at work can be the most difficult. Physical discomforts increase as your size does, and fatigue may really hound you. Your mood swings are hard to deal with. Be careful. In an effort to sustain your job performance and professional self, you may shortchange your partner, your family, and yourself. We all have limited emotional and physical resources. Are you expending most of yours on the job, being flexible, patient, noncomplaining, and polite, and then returning home depleted, a quick-tempered, sharp-tongued, negative pain in the neck? This might be a good time to leave. I confess this was true for me. My "good self" went to work, and my not-so-good self spent more time than I'd like to admit with my family. After all, they couldn't fire me. If you are under a lot of strain physically and emotionally, recognize that you may be placing an unfair burden on yourself and your family. Consider using some of your maternity leave before the baby's born or cutting back to part-time work if that's possible. Women I interviewed chose a variety of times to stop or ease off work. Laura, 35, remained active as a real-estate broker until the onset of labor. Elaine, 39, had periods of backache during her second trimester and was unable to do any desk work then, but she was able to resume work in her seventh month. Carmen, 41, taught school throughout the nine months and had a teaching assistant in place when it came time to leave; she adapted to late pregnancy by sitting at her desk or on a stool and cutting way back on standing at the chalkboard.

There are several things short of leaving your job you can do to ease pregnancy-related work problems. Outside of work, get plenty of sleep to combat fatigue, eat well, and exercise regularly. Be sure you're not carrying all or even most of the household chores; your partner must share these with you now. On the job, bring nutritious snacks to assuage your increased appetite and to infuse energy. Be sure your lunch is healthful, too. Move around during the day to keep circulation flowing in your legs. Keep your back supported. Prop your legs up while sitting at your desk, and flex your feet and ankles periodically. Arrange a way to sit down frequently if your job involves standing up for long periods of time. If feasible, catnaps and lying down on your left side can be beneficial. You'll have to cut back on heavy physical work late in pregnancy. Your center of gravity has shifted, and heavy lifting or strenuous activity carries a real risk of injury to strained and softened back, abdominal, and pelvic muscles and ligaments.

You may not think of your workplace as hazardous, but now that you're pregnant, you'll have to reassess it for possible danger. In fact, you should do this before you become pregnant so you and your partner can both avoid any known hazards. (For a discussion of teratogens and their effects on a fetus, see Chapter 7.) Are you, for instance, exposed to infectious diseases? Doctors, nurses, and schoolteachers frequently are. Do you work near a source of radiation? Dental workers, lab technicians, nurses, doctors, and nuclear power plant workers do. Are you exposed to toxic chemicals? Many, many workers are, among them beauticians, laundry or dry-cleaning employees, office personnel, and photo-lab workers. Do you come into daily contact with anesthesia? Operating room personnel and dental workers do. Substances that may not affect you normally can produce adverse reactions when you're pregnant.

A current controversy is whether video display terminals (VDTs) pose any hazard to a developing fetus. Experts say no, but studies are underway. It's a significant question because upwards of 10 million VDTs are now in use nationwide. While there is no scientific evidence that VDTs, through radiation or otherwise, cause miscarriages or birth defects, public concern has prompted epidemiological studies which may provide conclusive answers.

Guidelines on Pregnancy and Work, a booklet prepared by the American College of Obstetricians and Gynecologists and funded by the National Institute for Occupational Safety and Health, can help you assess the safety of your workplace. The ACOG guidelines list potentially harmful substances. Find out if you or your partner is being exposed to any of these substances at work or at home and discuss the situation with your practitioner. If your partner is being exposed, he may be bringing the toxin home to you. Unfortunately, thousands of new chemicals enter our environment annually, adding to the hundreds of thousands already there, so it's hard to keep up to date.

You are entitled to a change in job responsibilities to keep you from exposure to toxic substances during your pregnancy, and your employer can also insist on such a change. Some pregnant workers complain that they have been demoted or shifted to lower-paying jobs against their wishes by an employer claiming a risk of exposure when no significant risk actually existed. Whose right prevails in such cases is a murky area of the law.

Planning Your Leave

Many factors play a part in deciding when and for how long you should leave work. If you've been working for a long time, focusing your challenges and energies on your career, you may have no interest in stopping for very long. A woman over 35 is likely to have reached a level in her career that's rewarding both financially and emotionally. You can afford childcare. You can negotiate good benefits and flexible hours. You're accustomed to functioning as a professional person, and enjoy your status as one. You enjoy daily interaction with other adults in the workplace. You're accustomed to financial independence and do not want to rely on your husband for support.

On the other hand, your job may be simply too demanding to accommodate late pregnancy and parenthood. If you're an attorney who puts in standard 10- to 12-hour days plus weekends and frequent travel, how can you also care for an infant? No matter what position you hold, if your partner doesn't willingly share the responsibilities at home and/or you don't have paid help, you're not going to be very successful in both realms. Perhaps you're at a point in your career when you'd welcome the chance to take some time off or change course, develop new skills, explore different interests. Temporary or permanent retirement may be ideal for you now. You have a secure adult identity that can survive intact if you stop working. You may also feel it's important that you be the daily influence shaping your child's development. If it's to be your last child, you may want especially to involve yourself in her or his infancy and early development. But just remember that it can be very difficult for an older woman to reenter the job market.

"You take care of a baby? That's *all* you do?" Debbie, 36, vice president of marketing at a major cosmetics company, found this attitude in today's society rather daunting. Debbie had planned before the arrival of the baby to return to work immediately after the birth and had even gone so far as to schedule full-time sleep-in help. She and her husband, a medical doctor, could well afford the expense, and Debbie valued her independence. Unexpectedly, after delivery, she found herself experiencing emotions that would not allow her to leave the baby. But at the same time, she felt guilty about staying home. Her friends did not understand how Debbie could sacrifice so much. Debbie had to keep reminding herself that what she was doing was richly rewarding for both her and her child, and that she had a right to choose full-time mothering.

Remember when planning your leave that many women, like Debbie, enjoy being with their infants so much in the early months that they postpone a planned return to work. Be prepared to feel this way and try to make flexible leave plans beforehand. On the other hand, you may feel so confined after a few weeks that you're anxious to start at least part-time work as soon after delivery as possible. Astronaut Anna Fisher, for example, gave birth on a Friday and reported to work as usual on the following Monday. A lot of your challenges and energies may have gone into your career for a long time, in which case you could have a strong need to return to work soon. Be prepared for this possibility also, and plan accordingly.

In case you're feeling guilty about opting to go back to work, be aware that studies indicate children are happiest and best adjusted if their mothers enjoy what they are doing, whether that's working outside the home or devoting full time to childcare. Perhaps the costs of childcare don't leave much of your salary over. These costs won't continue indefinitely. Just treat them as a temporary business expense, to be shared by both parents. They are partly tax deductible. Do not fall into the trap of deducting those expenses from *your* salary and not your partner's or your combined salaries.

Because it's difficult to fit parenting into a 9-to-5 job, you and your partner might want to explore employment alternatives. Your current employer may offer these options, or you may find a different job with the right kind of hours. You may be able to do some of your work at home; propose this to your employer. Or perhaps you can develop an at-home business. Part-time work can be ideal in the late stages of pregnancy and after the baby is born, although it can be low-paying and benefit-poor. Job-sharing is another approach to part-time work in which you share your job as well as benefits with another person; this, too, can be ideal for a parent of small children. Susan and Ken did this on the campus of a small midwestern university. Both professors of English, they decided to accept a single tenured faculty position, splitting responsibilities, benefits, and salary. When Susan decided to become pregnant, her part-time work schedule was already operating, her childcare alternatives already built in.

Flextime and compressed time are both alternative forms of the 35- or 40-hour week. With compressed time, you work your

40 hours in fewer than five days, leaving at least three days a week off. With flextime, you choose which 8 hours you'll work in a day—say, from 6 A.M. to 2 P.M. There may be certain core hours you must include. You may also be allowed to trade benefits you don't want—such as medical insurance because your spouse already has it—for those you do—such as extra days off to spend with your child(ren). One innovative approach to making a traditionally inflexible, predominantly male field more adaptable is in use by a firm of lawyers in Washington, D.C., who hire themselves out to large, established law firms requiring extra help on a case-by-case basis. This allowed Rachel, a high-powered attorney, to continue practicing after she became pregnant and had a child, picking and choosing the cases she would work on. She also continued to draw a high salary, remained current in her field, and was able easily to integrate childcare with her working schedule.

Don't neglect the concept of househusbandry, even if you both hate the term. If this isn't a good time for a pause in your career, maybe it's just right for your partner. He can pursue new interests, acquire new skills, prepare for a career change instead of you. This hasn't become a common option yet, but at least it's no longer considered downright weird. Think about it. The arrangement has worked well for my friends Bob and Helen. Bob used the time to expand and rebuild their home, moving on to paid carpentry jobs when Samantha entered school. Helen continued her full-time career and further education as a nurse practitioner. Both parents are very satisfied with the results.

Planning for Childcare and Household Help

If you are going to continue working, you'll have to make childcare arrangements. Start early. You may be lucky and find someone or someplace right away, but chances are this will prove a challenge. You can't work if you don't have someone you can afford to care for your baby, and you won't work well if you don't have confidence that your baby is being well cared for. If you wait until the last minute or month, you may have to settle for an arrangement you consider less than adequate, which will make you feel guilty and anxious. One frustrated colleague insists the time to start searching for childcare is the day your pregnancy is confirmed! Set up childcare for the earliest date you expect to return to work. Should you decide or need to stay at home longer, you can make adjustments as required.

There are various childcare solutions to investigate. You may hire someone to come to your home and care for your baby. You may take your baby to another person's house. Relatives, if available, often work well in either of these situations. A woman (it never seems to be a man) caring for your baby in her home often has small children of her own, and she probably looks after several other children as well. She may or may not be licensed by your state as a daycare provider; either way, you'll need to check her house and her out thoroughly.

Group daycare centers are also available, and come in a number of forms: private run-for-profit, private nonprofit, government-funded. They have varying criteria and standards of care. Some have income ceilings; if you earn too much, they can't take your child. Some might not accept infants, and some may not be able to provide a lot of individual attention for your baby. The larger daycare centers are probably more appropriate for toddlers who can benefit from socializing. Almost all will be in great demand; many will have waiting lists. Employers sometimes provide on-site day care, which is ideally convenient but still rare. *American Baby* magazine reported in February 1984 that of companies it surveyed, 53% sponsor company sports teams, 48% support alcohol counseling for employees, and 1% provide childcare assistance. Citing those figures, you might canvass other parents among your co-workers and negotiate with your employer to set up a daycare facility at your workplace.

To locate childcare providers, ask friends, relatives, acquaintances, and other parents; call your state or local human services department and local daycare centers; check local nonprofit organizations like the YWCA or YMCA, churches, and colleges; read the classified ads in your local newspaper. This is not something you want to have to check out when you're the exhausted mother of a two-week-old. Do it now.

Even if you start well ahead of time, making childcare arrangements can be very frustrating. Searching for just the right person and situation may be like searching for the Holy Grail, and just as you think it's within your grasp it may slip away. That's what happened to Joyce, who started to plan her childcare months in advance, only to have each arrangement fall through. First she found a licensed daycare mother with a homey atmosphere, but an early-delivering mother took the open place that was to have been Joyce's. The licensed provider referred Joyce to another, unlicensed caretaker, who agreed to take on Joyce's baby but then changed her mind several weeks later. Entering her ninth month, Joyce began calling daycare centers near her and found them all full. She contacted state and local officials for a list of licensed home daycare providers, but no list was available. She got names of friends' babysitters; they were all booked. Joyce felt nervous and scared about her failure to make childcare arrangements as her due date approached. It was only after the birth of her son that Joyce finally found an available and acceptable daycare provider, whose facilities she felt were more than adequate—although not quite as good as what she would have held out for three months earlier.

Arranging for childcare isn't always this difficult, of course. When Marty was preparing for her first child at the age of 35, her husband Paul remembered a woman he'd grown up with who lived not far from Marty's office. The woman cared for a few children in her home, was happy to take on Marty and Paul's baby son, and is now caring for their infant daughter while the son attends nursery school.

Childcare is not the only help you must plan ahead for. Think about your needs while you're at home with your new baby. You can't care for a recently born infant, do all the other household chores, and remain well rested and relatively sane at the same time. In desperation, my husband and I once added up the hours required to bathe, feed, comfort, supply, and maintain a baby. It came out to 40 per week—and that was a good week, with a noncolicky baby. In the first weeks after delivery, by all means care for your baby yourself, but try to arrange for plenty of household help. This helps ward off postpartum depression, enables you to relax and enjoy spending time with your baby, and gets you back to work reasonably well rested. Either your spouse must run the house during this time, or you must get outside assistance from parents, brothers or sisters, inlaws, other relatives, or friends. Failing this you will need a paid housekeeper. Plan for this help, too, ahead of time.

Your Rights and Benefits

Before you make final arrangements for your maternity leave or job termination, you'll need to know what benefits your employer offers and what you are legally entitled to. An employer used to be able to discriminate grossly against pregnant employees, mandating early, unpaid maternity leave that also wiped out seniority rights. He used to be able to avoid providing disability medical insurance benefits for pregnancy—even when herniated males were paid as disabled workers and pregnant nonemployed wives were covered under their husbands' insurance. A 1978 amendment to the 1964 Civil Rights Act called the Pregnancy Discrimination Act plus several Supreme Court rulings in the 1970's finally established some legal rights for pregnant workers.

Basically, you cannot be treated differently than other workers because of your pregnancy. An employer may not refuse to hire or promote you because you are pregnant, nor can you be fired unless you're unable to perform your job. Maternity leave cannot be treated differently than other disability leave provided by the employer. This means you can't be forced to go on leave if you're still capable of doing your job; you can't be required to stay on leave if you're able to return to work, and you can't be called back before you're ready—unless all other temporarily disabled employees are subject to the same rules. You may not lose your seniority, job equivalent, or salary level after taking a leave if other workers returning from leave do not. Disability benefits and health plans must cover you if they cover other employees. You may not be denied unemployment compensation simply because you are pregnant; if you are able and willing to work, you qualify for it.

Note that your employer is not required to provide benefits if none exist for any workers. Also, the provisions of the 1978 act apply only to employers of 15 or more workers, or employers who deal with the federal government, so many women are still not guaranteed equal disability and health insurance benefits. Some states, though, have passed laws extending protection to employees of companies with less than 15 workers.

Find out what kind of leave is available from your employer. How long a disability leave can you take? Is it fully paid or partly paid? If your employer doesn't offer disability leave, can you take sick leave instead? If your employer doesn't offer any disability, your state may. If you use up your disability leave, can you continue on maternity leave? Is this paid or unpaid? Are there differences in benefits between managerial and nonmanagerial employees? Which do you qualify for? Inquire about other less obvious benefits. Does your partner's employer offer paternity leave? Is it paid or unpaid? Is any help available for childcare costs?

In planning your leave, remember that disabled means unable to work and so covers only the period just before you give birth and the period of recuperation afterward. If you choose to stay home with your baby much beyond that time, you may not be considered disabled and will have to negotiate a possible unpaid leave of absence. Clear this up with your employer in advance.

Your Health Insurance and Costs

Fortunately, we've progressed beyond the days when medical policies seemed designed to duck out from paying anything significant toward the cost of having a child. Group insurance plans offered by employers covered by the 1978 amendment cannot limit coverage for pregnancy unless all other coverages are similarly limited. You can't be required to pay your own insurance premiums, either, while you're on leave, unless all disabled workers must. However, if you're not covered by such a group policy, there may be substantial limitations on your maternity coverage. Read your policy, and find out.

First, figure out what expenses you're likely to incur during your pregnancy. With costs rising as rapidly as they are, it wouldn't be useful to estimate in this book what different providers will charge you; by the time it is printed, the figures would be out of date. One family practitioner I spoke to told me he had raised his total obstetrical fee by $100 recently only to have to increase it by another $100 the following month when his malpractice insurance premium doubled. If I had begun obstetrical care with him that day, I would have paid 35% more for his basic services than a woman who had started prenatal care two months earlier! With obstetrics being *the* high-risk specialty for malpractice, you can expect this trend to continue. Geographical factors also influence costs, with hospitals in urban areas generally charging more than those in rural locations; expenses in the Northeast are higher than in other regions.

Your pregnancy and childbirth may involve charges for a variety of the following items:

Doctors

— Attending physician; comprehensive fee, prenatal care through postpartum checkup

— Attending physician and/or surgeon: cesarean section

— Anesthesiologist

— Pediatrician's hospital care

— Attending physician or pediatrician: circumcision

Nurse–midwife

Genetic counselor

Classes

—Prepared childbirth

—Exercise

—Childcare

Tests, including:

—Pregnancy

—Blood and urine

—Alpha fetoprotein (AFP)

—Ultrasound

—Amniocentesis

Out-of-hospital birthing center

Hospital, including:

—Alternative birthing center

—Room and board, maternal

—private

—semiprivate

—Nursery

—regular

—special care

—Labor room

—Delivery room

—Fetal monitoring

—Lab tests

—Medications

There are several twists you need to be aware of in calculating your expected coverage. Your insurance plan will probably be divided into hospital and medical or major medical coverage. Hospital benefits cover charges for services in the hospital such as medications, diagnostic tests, and room and board. The latter may be completely covered or covered only up to a maximum daily charge, over which you pay the rest. Blue Cross is the most common hospital policy.

Medical coverage like Blue Shield and/or major medical pays doctors' fees—sometimes all, sometimes a percentage, sometimes a fixed amount for fixed services, especially surgery. Examine your policy to see what portion of your doctors' fees is covered. Figure out if diagnostic tests are paid for if they're performed in your doctor's office or on an outpatient basis at the hospital. You don't want a $600 amniocentesis done at your doctor's office if your medical insurance only pays when it's done in-hospital. Genetic counseling may be covered if it's part of the amniocentesis procedure, but not if it's done independently.

If your policy covers "complications of pregnancy," find out what these are; your insurance company will have its own definitions, and it's nice to know you'll be covered if your doctor orders a week in the hospital to help avert preterm labor. Are you choosing a nurse–midwife as your birth attendant and/ or an out-of-hospital birthing center as your birth setting? These may or may not be covered by your health insurance. Be sure you don't run afoul of any waiting period on a new policy if you were pregnant when your coverage began. Also find out when and to whom benefits are paid—your insurer may pay you after you've paid the provider or, more likely it will pay the provider directly, who will in turn bill you for the balance. If the hospital is aware of an uninsured balance, it may, outrageously, attempt not to discharge you until this sum is paid. I know from first-hand experience that this can happen. It's not legal—leave anyway, without paying. Also be sure to leave by check-out time to avoid being charged for an extra day.

One thing you must be certain of is that your infant is covered from the moment of birth. Neonatal nursery fees can be crushing if not paid by an insurer. Some plans don't cover the baby until it's 15 to 31 days old, leaving the first critical period, when expenses can be the greatest, uncovered. Other plans will pay the amount over the regular-care daily nursery charge if the baby has a birth problem that meets the insurer's guidelines. Almost all states now require that newborns be covered from birth in all *new* health insurance policies. If your policy was written before your state's law went into effect, or by a company in an uncovered state, your infant may still be uncovered. Check this very carefully, with your employer or insurance commissioner, and get some sort of coverage if you don't have any. Who can afford $20,000 to $200,000 in medical bills?

If both you and your husband work, you may both have insurance policies with your respective employers. Check the policies to see if one provides better maternity coverage than the other. Use the second to take care of any balance due. It's very unlikely you could collect more than 100% of your medical expenses; policies usually have a provision to prevent this. You might find you have significant overlapping coverage and you might want to consolidate this into a single policy. But if, in choosing to do this, you select your spouse's policy and he then leaves his job and thus his group, you'll both have to convert to a new contract and possibly a new insurer. If your employers are paying all or most of your insurance premiums, it's probably safest and easiest to stick with the double coverage.

Knowing what employee and health insurance benefits to expect makes it possible to plan financially for your baby's arrival. You'll know what your family income will be, and you can make payment arrangements for balances due ahead of time to fit your budget. While you're calculating, you can also figure in other baby-related costs that will arise during and shortly after pregnancy. These might include:

Maternity clothes
Baby equipment, such as:
  —crib
  —dresser
  —changing table
  —backpack and sling
  —car seat
  —stroller
  —toys
Baby-care items, such as:
  —diapers
  —bottles
  —formula
  —vitamin drops

Baby clothing
Childcare
Housekeeping help
Pediatrician's fees

Understanding the financial requirements may help you decide on the timing and length of your maternity leave. It may give you something concrete to fuss about, but at least it'll relieve you of unknown financial anxiety throughout your pregnancy!

CHAPTER 10

PREGNANCY AFTER 40: SPECIAL CONSIDERATIONS

Since childbearing through the mid or late 30's has become increasingly common, the question inevitably arises: If it's relatively safe to have a baby at 39, why not at 40, or 41, or later? Interestingly, *Harper's Bazaar* ran an article in September 1979 entitled "Childbirth After 30." Two years later, in September 1981, the topic was "Childbirth After 40."

Medical Considerations

The majority of doctors, when asked their opinion on the matter, tell the healthy woman in her early 40's considering childbearing to go ahead with it but to monitor her pregnancy closely. This means paying special attention to prenatal care. From a physiological standpoint, the risks are more appreciable for a woman of this age. This holds true for the mother having a first baby, a subsequent baby, or, as is more often the case, the last baby.

Before discussing these increased risks for the over-40 mother, it is important to reiterate that perhaps the most troubling aspect of having a baby at this time of life is the difficulty of getting pregnant in the first place. This is because, unfortunately, all age-related fertility problems have had more time to develop—diminished quantity and quality of eggs, skipped ovulation and reproductive system disorders. In short, becoming pregnant is much less easily accomplished. This is also true for women between 35 and 40, but the risk of infertility increases noticeably after 40, perhaps by 50%. Now there isn't much, if any, time for fertility treatments. Most women cease menstrual function entirely between 45 and 55 years of age. To further hinder conception, couples in their 40's generally have intercourse less often than younger couples, although this may not be true for the over-40 couple trying to accomplish pregnancy. A bright spot: there is no known appreciable drop in the over-40 male's ability to produce sufficient sperm to achieve fertilization.

In second place for the most troubling aspect about having a post-40 baby is the possibility of bearing a child with a major birth defect—for this is more of a hazard for a woman over 40 than for one between 35 and 39. The amniocentesis study whose results are charted in Chapter 6 found that 4.8% of the 40-plus mothers had abnormalities, while only 1.4% of the mothers 35 to 39 did. The incidence of major birth defects in live births also charted in Chapter 6 rose from 1.7% among women 35 to 39 to 3.1% for mothers 40 to 44. Women 45 and over experienced a rate of 7.6%. The risks appear greatest for chromosome abnormalities, especially Down's syndrome, and congenital heart disease. The incidence of Down's jumps from 1 out of 400 at age 35 to 1 out of 105 at age 40 to 1 out of 35 at age 44.

Expressed as percentages, these risks may not seem high. Nevertheless, they illustrate why the use of amniocentesis—an important tool to the pregnant woman over 35—approaches critical proportions for the woman over 40. As discussed in Chapter 6, the reduction in risk of severe birth defects for mothers over 40 with full use of available detection and intervention/termination techniques is 68%.

Unfortunately, researchers found in 1980 that pregnant women aged 40 or more do not use prenatal chromosomal diagnosis more frequently than women 35 to 36, despite the fact that the older women are at five times greater risk. In some areas the use of amniocentesis even *dropped* among women over 40 as compared with women in their later 30's!

Since women over 40 are much more likely to conceive a defective fetus, it isn't surprising that these women have a higher abortion rate than their younger counterparts. The Center for Disease Control, in its 1978 Surveillance Abortion Report, found 788 elective abortions per 1,000 live births among women aged 40 or more. This is a much higher figure than that for women 35 to 39, who had 435 per 1,000. While the statistics do not indicate how many of these abortions were for medical reasons, it is likely that most occurred at the wish of the mother.

Women who conceive when they are 40-plus are also more likely to have a spontaneous abortion than women 35 to 39, who themselves are at three times greater risk for miscarriage than women in their 20's. Though it is not known for sure, it is likely that a fair percentage of these abortions occur because of defects in the embryo or early fetus. Most of these spontaneous abortions take place before a woman knows she is pregnant or within the first few months of pregnancy.

The potential for complications of full-term pregnancy increases with age, so it is highest for the oldest members of the obstetric population—women 40 and over. In medical terms, you're a "very elderly gravida" at this age! The mother's body, simply as a function of age, has had more time to develop problems. The pregnant 40-plus woman is definitely more likely to have high blood pressure, sometimes with toxemia developing, and pregnancy-related diabetes. Urinary tract infections and benign tumors are also more common, as are premature contractions. Of course, every additional year means additional exposure to all the environmental hazards. Postmaturity, a condition in which an overdue baby is no longer adequately supported by the placenta, is more common in first-time over-40 mothers.

The outcome of over-40 pregnancies has been widely researched. The results are somewhat conflicting. A study reported by Dr. Sidney Kane in 1967, mentioned in Chapter 6, is still commonly referred to in spite of the years that have elapsed. Kane found a much higher incidence of high-risk deliveries for women over 40, but the increase was from 0.4% for 25- to 29-year-olds to only 1.4% for women 40 to 45, which still amounts to a very small number of women.

Virtually all studies report that many more cesarean sections are performed on older mothers, with the rate quoted as being highest for women over 40. In the Kane study it rose as high as 35% for women ages 41 and 42. A large Finnish study of mothers 40 and over published in the *International Journal of Gynaecology and Obstetrics*, Volume 19, in 1981 found a whopping cesarean rate of 47% for first-time mothers; for all women in the group, the rate was a still-high 17%.

Does a child born to an over-40 mother have as good a chance of survival as a younger woman's child? It seems so. There has been some documentation of more perinatal deaths among infants born to women over 40, but other figures contradict this. A woman over 40 is more likely to deliver her baby prematurely. However, the Kane study found that the survival rate of these infants, along with those born to women from 35 to 39, was no different from the survival rate of other babies. The 1981 Finnish report confirmed this and, in fact, found no difference between the survival rates for all infants born to women 40 and over and those of younger women's infants. While the baby of an over-40 mother is a bit more likely to develop problems such as high bilirubin levels or infection, most of these conditions are quite amenable to treatment, and the infant can be expected to develop normally.

The authors of the Finnish report studying only women 40 or more mentioned some interesting pluses. First-time mothers tended generally to be in better health than those with previous pregnancies, and had less high blood pressure. The great majority of mothers with chronic disease diagnosed at the outset had "uneventful" pregnancies and did well postpartum. Surprisingly, no greater risk of either prematurity or a low birth weight was found for the over-40 mother, nor were there more anomalies. These authors concluded that the health and life of the over-40 woman are not endangered by pregnancy. They also concluded that risks to the newborn could be lowered to nearly the level of younger mothers' babies if prenatal care, labor, and delivery were carefully monitored and managed. This is the same outcome as for women 35 to 39.

Social and Emotional Considerations

Most women who become pregnant after 40 are not first-time mothers. If the pregnancy is unplanned, it can cause quite an emotional quandary. Abortion will probably be seriously considered. A woman who has children often finds it difficult to terminate a pregnancy. She has experienced the delightfully individual personality and potential each new birth represents. On the other hand, she may not relish starting over with a newborn. Her children may all be established in school and old enough to require little after-school care. She may have reentered the job market or professional world and begun to place her own career goals in a priority position. Her husband may share her ambivalence. Possibly, he's glad that his partner is at last less childcare-oriented, and able once again to participate in activities with him. A new baby will complicate that interaction. Under these circumstances, deciding whether or not to proceed with the pregnancy can be especially difficult.

First-time parents over 40 are usually delighted. They have to keep in mind that it's okay to have only one child. A woman who has her first child after her 40th birthday will no doubt weigh very carefully the option of having a second. There simply may not be time to have more, especially if she and her partner would prefer to space children by several years, as many childcare experts now suggest.

Divorce and remarriage contribute to a growing number of new fathers in their 40's and 50's, many with grown or nearly grown children from the first marriage. These men generally express great satisfaction with the new parental role. Tom, 51 and father of a 2-year-old son, is typical. In contrast to his earlier fathering which began when he was 29, Tom doesn't let his work routine keep him from spending evenings and weekends with his toddler. He feels much more involved with his young son's development and is experiencing a more sharing relationship. Tom's teenage son loves teaching new skills to his baby brother and is learning to assume a nurturing role. Tom's enjoyment of his new child enables him to laugh when he's asked about his "grandchild."

On the personal side, my second child was born when I was 40. After researching this topic, I can see that I had a pretty typical 40-plus pregnancy. My husband and I thought about an abortion early in the pregnancy, which was unplanned; a new baby seemed very difficult to integrate into our lives. I was awfully tired during that pregnancy (more so than in my first, when I was 36); I worked more than I would have liked and was troubled by contractions during the last 10 weeks. I did have a touch of sugar in my urine which went away. The minor problems our son, Jamie, experienced were typical, too. He was a little smaller than average and required some treatment for high bilirubin but was and is a very healthy baby. My husband and I are now delighted to be 41-year-old parents of a 1-year-old.

All things considered, the pregnant woman over 40 who decides to take her pregnancy to term and who is faithful to good prenatal care has a very good chance of remaining healthy herself and having a healthy, normal baby—just like her slightly younger 35- to 39-year-old sisters. The key for both classes of women seems to be good prenatal care. Seek it out early in your over-40 pregnancy and maintain it throughout. The reward? In one woman's words, "Being a new parent at 42 is tiring, complicated, life-transforming, and the most satisfying thing I've ever done."

CHAPTER 11

AFTERMATH

Once you have given birth and embarked on the lengthy process of parenthood, your life will be permanently altered. While it's not the function of this book to counsel you on childcare and parenting, no volume on pregnancy is complete without a discussion of the immediate postpartum period—the first few months after delivery, which can be called the "fourth trimester" of pregnancy. Two major constellations of changes affect you during this time. Profound physical changes occur quite rapidly as you return to a prepregnant condition. Equally profound changes occur to alter the emotional structure of your life.

Physical Events Postpartum

While you will shed a lot of your extra bulk and fluid during delivery, your body will take some time to return to a completely nonpregnant state. Immediately after delivery of the placenta, the uterus begins to contract, which you will feel as cramping after-pains. Since the uterus doesn't shed its extra muscle and shrink to its prepregnant size (almost) for six weeks, you can't expect a perfectly flat abdomen for at least that long. As the uterus contracts down ("involutes"), its lining regenerates, taking about three weeks to do so. The site where the placenta detached from also heals, in about six weeks. While these changes are occurring, blood is discharged from the uterus through the vagina. This fluid is called lochia, and you can expect it to continue flowing for up to four weeks after delivery. It may be somewhat heavy for the first few days, but then will lighten up considerably, until it's just spotting. Lochia will be bright red at first, then become paler and finally, yellowish or brownish. You'll need to wear sanitary pads or liners until the discharge stops. Should you pass large clots, bleed extremely heavily at the outset, or resume heavy bleeding after a period of light discharge, notify your practitioner immediately.

The cervix and vagina return to their prepregnant condition in about three weeks. If you had an episiotomy, the stitches should heal completely after that time, although they may cause some pain and swelling before then. If the stitches become uncomfortable, sitz baths (soaking in warm water) or soothing cream can help.

Blood volume drops rapidly in the first few days after delivery, and accumulated tissue fluids also are expelled. This results in temporarily increased urination, possibly accompanied by increased thirst. Just think of the extra trips to the bathroom as a welcome way to shed more of your excess weight. If the bladder or the urethra was bruised during delivery, you may have trouble urinating for a day or two. An epidural, too, can inhibit bladder function for several hours. Both conditions usually clear themselves up. Bowel function normally resumes spontaneously after delivery; sometimes it is helped along by a small dose of laxative. To avoid constipation during the first week or two when you're less active than usual, continue to follow the pregnancy recommendations in Chapter 4.

Your heartrate and respiration also return to normal levels within a few months after delivery. The dark pigmentation around your nipples or running down your abdomen will clear away, and any stretch marks will fade gradually to the silvery whitish tone they'll keep permanently.

Changes in your breasts will vary, depending on whether or not you're breastfeeding. Milk production begins within three days of delivery. If you don't breastfeed, your breasts may feel uncomfortably full and sore for a while. Wear a tight bra, apply ice packs, and *don't* press any milk out of your breasts; this will just stimulate production of more milk. If you do breastfeed, wear a supporting bra night and day, and keep the nipples clean by rinsing with water. Empty the breasts at each feeding to prevent engorgement—swelling and hardness.

The return of ovulation and menstruation varies greatly with the individual. After delivery of the placenta, the elevated levels of the pregnancy hormones fall abruptly, permitting renewed release of the hormones that stimulate ovulation and uterine bleeding. You may resume ovulation as soon as four weeks after delivery; many women do by six weeks, and most by twelve weeks. A breastfeeding mother maintains exceptionally high levels of the hormone prolactin, which suppresses ovulation, so she may not ovulate or menstruate while she is breastfeeding. However, don't count on breastfeeding as a safe method of contraception—it isn't! No matter how you're feeding your baby, you may ovulate *before* your first postpregnancy menstrual period, so contraception at all times is an absolute must when you and your partner reinitiate sexual intercourse. Menstruation, when it does occur, may be quite heavy at first. About six weeks after delivery you'll return to your practitioner for a final, postpartum checkup to be sure your physical recovery from pregnancy is complete and normal.

Personal Care Postpartum

Whether you stay at your birth center 12 hours or 3 days, you'll be urged to start "early ambulation"—getting up and around soon and often after delivery. This is important to regain muscle tone, stimulate circulation in the legs, encourage uterine shrinkage and drainage, and minimize bowel and bladder problems. It will also make you feel less like an invalid and more like a healthy person who's in charge of her situation. No wonder our mothers were virtual invalids after giving birth— they were kept in bed in the hospital for two weeks and came home, inevitably, weak and shaky.

Once you're home, though, don't confuse "early ambulation" with a resumption of your normal level of activity. Your uterus has not healed yet; excessive activity or strain can lead to excessive vaginal bleeding. Just as you had to adjust to the physical strains of pregnancy, you'll now have to readjust to your prepregnant center of gravity and compensate for those overstretched baby-supporting muscles, ligaments, and joints. Don't strain or push, don't lift anything heavy, and don't run up and down stairs. In fact, avoid stairs; when you must use them, go up and down very slowly. You'll be even less able to be physically active if you're recovering from a particularly difficult delivery or a cesarean section.

The main consideration in these early months is *rest*, which, granted, is extremely hard to get. All the factors are present to plunge you into exhaustion. You start parenthood extremely tired out from the exertions of labor and delivery. Caring for a new baby is incredibly demanding, and you can't bolster your resources with uninterrupted sleep. The problem is multiplied if you have other small children to care for. If you try to maintain a normal schedule of activity, there's no way to make up for it at night. You simply must plan on and take frequent rest breaks during the day. Limiting visitors for the first few weeks is a good idea, too. Inadequate rest will affect you psychologically and physically, so that you won't be able to nurse or care for your baby well. Fatigue is the enemy of all new mothers, but it seems particularly troublesome to older women, so take extra precautions to maintain your energy level.

Your birth center and practitioner will give you instructions about personal care for the first few weeks after delivery. There will be special ones for nursing mothers; see the section later in this chapter on breastfeeding. In general, showers rather than baths will be advised for the first week or two. The area around the episiotomy should be washed with soap and water several times a day and after bowel movements. Don't abandon your well-balanced diet now; it's needed to promote rapid recovery, avoid anemia, and bolster energy levels. Your practitioner may recommend that you continue vitamin and iron supplements for a while, too. Even if you gained excess weight during the pregnancy, don't rush to shed it all in the first few postpartum weeks; give yourself several months to get back to your normal weight. This does not mean that you will have recovered your muscle tone.

One of the most difficult adjustments postpartum is the discovery that you haven't shrunk back to your prepregnancy size right after delivery. Walking down the hospital corridor the day after my first child was born, I was dismayed when a cheeky young nurse's aide looked at my stomach and giggled, "Did you have your baby yet?" Don't be shocked or discouraged when you don't fit right back into your normal clothes and still have to wear loose-fitting garments for a while—even possibly, god forbid, some of those maternity clothes you thought you'd never have to look at again after you gave birth. To hasten the return of your former wardrobe and to soften any age-related difficulty in regaining muscle tone, fix your mind on faithful performance of your postpartum exercise routine, which it's important to initiate as soon after delivery as possible. Sad to say, while nature will shrink your uterus, it won't flatten out your abdomen—only you can do that, through exercise. It took nine months to grow to predelivery size, and it can take that long to get back to your original shape.

What exercises do you do? First, you'll probably be given a series of mild strengthening exercises by your hospital or birthing center to do for the first few days. Once you're home, your choices are similar to those outlined in Chapter 7. Books like the ones cited there outline postpartum as well as prenatal exercise routines. Classes are a great way to get yourself out of the house; the YMCA's "You & Me, Baby" offers exercises to shape you up *and* to stimulate your baby. You do need clearance from your practitioner for whatever exercise routine you adopt.

Sexual Relations Postpartum

As your body begins to recover, you and your partner will most likely become increasingly interested in resuming sexual relations. Your practitioner will probably have given you specific recommendations about when you can reinitiate intercourse. It's generally advised that you wait until all perineal tearing and suturing have healed, the cervix and vagina have returned to normal, and the lochia (discharge) has become minimal, all of which may take about three weeks. Some practitioners want you to wait until after the six-week checkup to engage in sex.

You may not be too eager to resume intercourse soon after delivery. This is perfectly normal. Relations between you and your partner should return to prepregnancy levels by the end of three months or so. Masters and Johnson report in *Human Sexual Response* that nursing mothers experience significantly higher levels of sexual interest in the early postpartum months than nonbreastfeeders.

Independent of desire, you might find intercourse uncomfortable at first. This can be caused by decreased vaginal lubrication and vaginal distention in the first few weeks after delivery; the lochia can cause postcoital irritation, too. These conditions will clear up soon, so if intercourse is initially uncomfortable, wait a few days before trying again.

Psychological Adjustments

Considerable as the physical changes you have undergone are, they are by no means the most profound you'll undergo postpartum. The psychological and lifestyle aftereffects are immense. Some of these have already been discussed. Although you know intellectually it's absurd, you get the feeling that your baby will always be this tiny and utterly dependent. You feel isolated and trapped while surrounded by this crushing responsibility; you're housebound and feel cut off from the outside world. You may not have been prepared for your prenatal support system to vanish abruptly, may not have realized how much you relied on your childbirth and exercise classes, which now have ceased, and on your practitioner, whom you won't see until the six-week postpartum checkup. You scarcely know your pediatrician, who in any case is concerned with the baby, not you.

Add to this the abrupt postdelivery drop in hormone levels that returns you to a state of "emotional lability"—those wildly fluctuating mood swings—and one moment you're drenched in love and pride toward your child, the next you're sobbing with frustration. You used to be in control of your life, and now you feel totally out of it. Is there any wonder most women experience a period of postpartum blues, or mild depression? Clinical depression calls for counseling treatment, but the common blues of the first few weeks usually pass within a relatively short time and can be moderated or perhaps warded off with some informed self-help.

Rest can combat depression. It can supplement the absence of pregnancy's hormonal glow, which disappears upon delivery, and it can make you feel better about your appearance. Make your baby's pattern yours. If he or she tends to sleep all day and then cranks up when the sun goes down, you'll have to do the same at first in order to get adequate rest. The child will eventually settle into a more "normal" pattern, although it's hard to believe that right now.

Another way to counteract postdelivery stress is to treat yourself—for instance, to a new hairdo or a few splurge dinners out with your partner. Such indulgences may do wonders for your morale—and his, too. Once you are able to get out of the house a bit, do so. Postnatal exercise groups at the YWCA, for example, are a good place to meet women with whom you share something in common. They can relieve your feelings of alienation and provide you with someone other than your partner to confide in. At home, be lenient with yourself; read a book or take a hot bath instead of vacuuming the floor or washing the dishes. Have your helper and/or your partner do some things just for you, like fixing a special lunch or laundering some of your hand-washables.

You should work out feelings of anxiety, depression, and unhappiness, which are normal and understandable, with your partner, so he knows what's happening. You might share these and not realize it. He, too, is bound to be affected by reduced sleep, by the upheaval of established home routines and your recovery needs, by the pressure of ever-present childcare tasks, by the actual assumption of the planned-for new identity, by sexual desires and anxieties and by a burdensome feeling of responsibility. Just as when you were pregnant it was important to communicate, you don't want a separation to develop during this postpartum period from lack of connectedness. Remind each other to concentrate on the immediate present rather than dwell on the enormity of the total responsibility.

Be sure to integrate the baby into your family rather than transfer your attention from your partner to the infant. Under the pressure of new motherhood, a woman can tend to put the baby first, with herself as a poor second and her partner virtually out of the running. Fortunately, men today actively participate in childcare (this is especially true of older new fathers), so you and your partner can share time together as you share baby-maintenance tasks. This also assures that your partner won't feel left out or displaced by his own child. Furthermore, if he shares the responsibility, it will become a joint venture and you won't resent having to carry the whole burden.

Be sure, too, to leave baby and father alone together at times, so your partner has a chance to gain confidence in his ability to care for the infant without your instant backup. You still need time, however, to interact as an adult twosome rather than always as parents and child. Consciously make time for this in your daily lives, even though it may seem especially difficult in the early months after delivery.

Breast and Bottle Feeding

A large part of the early postpartum routine revolves around feeding your baby. A new baby doesn't have a large stomach capacity and so must nurse often, even at intervals during the night. Part of the postdelivery adjustment is getting to know your baby's needs—how often and how much she or he needs to be fed. Your birth center and your pediatrician will give you detailed information on infant feeding and on the pros and cons of breast and bottle feeding. We'll look at a few particular considerations here.

Breastfeeding does have certain advantages, such as emotional satisfaction for both mother and infant, temporary transfer of maternal immunities to the baby, and provision of a nonallergenic "perfect" food. Of special interest to you as an older mother is the fact that breastfeeding will help you get back into shape faster; nursing releases the hormone oxytocin, which stimulates the uterus to contract and shrink back to its normal size. Breastfeeding is also more convenient in the sense that you don't have to fuss with bottles, nipples, formula, and sterilizing, which is particularly gratifying at 2 A.M. on a cold night. Breastfeeding is also more economical, since there's nothing extra to buy except several nursing bras and a bit more food for you.

However, breastfeeding is not more convenient if you return to work soon after your baby's birth. If you miss a feeding, your baby will have to be given a substitute bottle, filled either with formula or your own milk expressed earlier with a breast pump. Your breasts will leak milk at unpredictable times, which can be disconcerting in a board meeting; nursing mothers must wear shields inside their bras to avoid staining. If you don't nurse or pump thoroughly at regular intervals, your milk supply will dwindle. Many mothers do successfully work full-time and breastfeed, but it's not easy. Your employer may not be supportive; a maternity nurse I know was asked by her supervisor if she was pumping breast milk for later feeding on hospital time or on her own unpaid time. You might consider breastfeeding while you're home on maternity leave and then gradually weaning the baby when you return to full-time work.

Breastfeeding also requires a continuation of the special attention to diet and ingestion of drugs that was necessary during pregnancy. Many substances pass through your breast milk to your baby, and vitamin content of human milk is largely dependent on a mother's daily diet. Because of the nutrients needed to sustain your baby, and the energy consumed to produce the milk, you expend an extra 600 to 800 calories daily when breastfeeding, and your specific nutrient requirements are also increased, as shown by the chart in Chapter 7. Only a part of the fat deposits you accumulated during pregnancy will be shed if you breastfeed; the rest are needed for milk production. You may not, therefore, get back to your prepregnancy weight until after your baby's weaned. Some nursing mothers, however, find their weight melts away.

Parents sometimes feel that breastfeeding interferes with the father's ability to become intimately involved with the nurturing of his child—a particular concern of the older father. Actually, though, there are many activities surrounding the actual suckling which the father can take charge of. He can respond to the baby's cries for food, pick up, change, comfort, and burp the infant, decide whether the baby needs feeding or some other form of attention. He can be the one to get up at 3 A.M., tend to and bring the baby to the mother in bed for nursing, or even give the infant a bottle so the mother can continue to sleep.

Older mothers are more likely to breastfeed than bottle feed. This seems somewhat paradoxical, since most over-35 mothers also work outside the home, making breastfeeding inconvenient. The best guess of those who've observed this characteristic is that it's part of the older mother's total preparation for the best possible pregnancy and parenting. Today's wisdom is that breastfeeding is most beneficial to a baby, so the older mother wholeheartedly commits herself to that form of feeding regardless of convenience factors.

Breast or bottle, paid employment or full-time mothering, first child or last—childbearing after 35 is challenging and absorbing. Acceptance and medical management of "elderly" pregnancy has come a long way since my friend Will's mother experienced a mysterious abdominal complaint in 1950 at the age of 43 after seven years of childless marriage. Treated by her family doctor for months with a variety of medications to cure the suspected tumor, the woman—and her doctor—finally grasped what the problem was when a neighbor listened to the details of the case, looked at her friend, and declared, "Mildred, you're pregnant!" The obvious diagnosis had been overlooked for seven months because of Mildred's age and previous childlessness.

A similar incident would be unthinkable today. Neither prospective parents nor obstetricians would ignore the possibility of pregnancy for a premenopausal woman simply because she was over 35 or over 40. If you are an over-35 childbearer or plan to be one you can feel secure in the knowledge that you're part of a large and building wave—women who are no longer pioneers but settlers. There is, today, an array of medical services to protect and promote your pregnancy and a society that is accepting and welcoming. When your offspring reaches childbearing age, he or she will probably look back at the questions raised today by over-35 pregnancy and ask, "What was all the fuss about?"

INDEX